汉英
对照

口岸卫生检疫
实用手册

AN ESSENTIAL MANUAL FOR
HEALTH QUARANTINE AT PORTS

黎 文◎编著

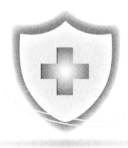

U0313319

中国海关出版社有限公司

中国·北京

图书在版编目（CIP）数据

口岸卫生检疫实用手册：汉英对照/黎文编著．

—北京：中国海关出版社有限公司，2022.6

ISBN 978 - 7 - 5175 - 0582 - 2

Ⅰ.①口…　Ⅱ.①黎…　Ⅲ.①国境检疫—卫生检疫—中国—手册—汉、英　Ⅳ.①R185.3-62

中国版本图书馆 CIP 数据核字（2022）第 099478 号

口岸卫生检疫实用手册

KOUAN WEISHENG JIANYI SHIYONG SHOUCE

作　　者：黎　文

策划编辑：景小卫

责任编辑：景小卫　刘白雪

出版发行：中国海关出版社有限公司

社　　址：北京市朝阳区东四环南路甲 1 号　　　　邮政编码：100023

网　　址：www. hgcbs. com. cn

编 辑 部：01065194242-7527（电话）

发 行 部：01065194221/4238/4246/5127/7543（电话）

社办书店：01065195616（电话）
　　　　　https://weidian. com/? userid = 319526934(网址)

印　　刷：北京鑫益晖印刷有限公司　　　　　　　经　　销：新华书店

开　　本：710mm×1000mm　1/16

印　　张：13.75　　　　　　　　　　　　　　　字　　数：200 千字

版　　次：2022 年 6 月第 1 版

印　　次：2022 年 6 月第 1 次印刷

书　　号：ISBN 978 - 7 - 5175 - 0582 - 2

定　　价：56.00 元

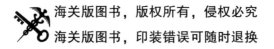

谨以此书致敬奋战在一线"抗疫"的逆行者们

THIS BOOK IS DEDICATED TO THOSE WHO
ARE FIGHTING AGAINST COVID-19
ON THE FRONTLINES

前　言
Preface

　　自 2020 年新冠肺炎疫情席卷全球以来，世界卫生组织（WHO）宣布全球进入公共卫生紧急状态，直至今天人类尚未摆脱这种状态，疫情仍在全球持续蔓延，对全球公共卫生安全造成严重的冲击，抗击疫情已成为全人类共同的使命。新冠肺炎作为一种新发传染病，在全球高位流行，新冠病毒持续变异，变异毒株在世界流行较为广泛。世界卫生组织数据显示，截至 2022 年 3 月 31 日，全球新冠肺炎累计报告确诊病例 4.87 亿例，死亡 616.2 万例。

　　针对疫情，全球各国和地区采取了不同的"抗疫"措施。现在看来，过早"解封"将导致疫情反弹，如欧美国家 2021 年 9 月"解封"后就出现了第四轮疫情传播高峰。新冠肺炎疫情发生以来，我国政府始终坚持人民至上、生命至上，坚持"外防输入、内防反弹"，坚持"动态清零"总方针，因时因势不断调整防控措施，疫情防控取得重大战略成果，最大限度减少了人群感染，维护了人民生命安全和身体健康。两年多来，我国战胜了武汉疫情，迅速扑灭数十起局部散发病例和聚集性疫情，有效减少了死亡病例，经济表现居于全球前列。

　　目前，我国"外防输入、内防反弹"的防控形势依然严峻，面临国外疫情随解封反弹、病毒变异传播力增强等形势，口岸"外防输入"的工作压力越来越大。为进一步做好新冠肺炎疫情防控，巩固常态化疫情防控，深圳海关根据口岸重点关切，及时有效、动态调整疫情防控措施，第一时间成立了疫情防控指挥部及相应的疫情防控专业小组，以便现场引导出入境旅客健康申报、入境外交人员卫生检疫等相关工作。为配合提升一线海关关员的执法能力和关员的外语水平，笔者作为深圳湾海关疫情防控翻译小组组长，结合口岸关注的传染病、口岸卫生检疫流程，利用业余时间加班加点，完成了本书的中英双语编写工作。

本书共分五章，分别为口岸重点关注的传染病、旅客通关与健康防护、口岸卫生检疫场景表达、口岸卫生检疫相关规范文件、口岸疫情防控文摘。笔者参照《口岸新型冠状病毒肺炎卫生检疫操作指南》《新型冠状病毒肺炎卫生检疫引导用语参考规范》等文件，搜集大量相关网站和国内外报刊资料，对口岸重点关注的传染病进行介绍，对口岸卫生检验流程进行梳理并整理成场景式对话，同时收集整理了疫情防控工作中涉及的法律法规等，以汉英对照的方式汇编成书。为方便读者更好地理解本书英文内容，笔者在相关章节后面均附上了名词解释。此外，为增加本书的实用性，笔者在附录部分收集了出入境健康申明卡、申报指南等供读者参考。

本书旨在为一线关员与出入境旅客现场交流、旅客通关及入境外交人员的卫生检疫提供指导和帮助，具有较强的操作性和实用性。

在编写本书过程中，笔者得到了深圳海关领导和同事的大力指导和帮助，特别是深圳海关卫生检疫处吴迪迪、罗伟权、曲鑫、仲媛等对本书专业内容的把关和审核，法规处同事对本书法规内容的审核，以及深圳湾海关疫情防控翻译小组成员前期部分资料整理等，笔者在此表示诚挚的谢意！

由于编写时间仓促，水平有限，书中难免有疏漏之处，欢迎读者批评指正。

黎　文

2022 年 5 月

目　录

Contents

1 口岸重点关注的传染病
Infectious Diseases of Particular Concern at Ports

导读：传染病是由各种病原体引起的能在人与人、动物与动物或人与动物之间相互传播的一类疾病。传染病对人类的生存和健康有很大危害。早在古代就出现了包括天花、恶性疟疾、麻疹、腺鼠疫、肺鼠疫等能够强烈致死的人畜共患病。

过去十多年里，我们见证了诸多流行病的暴发：2009 年的甲型 H1N1 流感、2014 年的基孔肯雅热、2015 年的寨卡病毒病以及 2014 年在西非暴发流行的埃博拉病毒病。此外，2002—2003 年的传染性非典型肺炎（SARS）几乎造成了大流行，2012 年的中东呼吸综合征首次在阿拉伯被发现。

当前全球贸易高位运行，人员跨境流动频繁，重大烈性传染病跨境传播概率和暴发流行风险与日俱增。为巩固常态化疫情防控，适应当前全球传染病流行复杂态势，有效防止传染病传入传出，维护国门和人民健康安全，必须科学规范口岸传染病的卫生检疫工作。

口岸重点关注的传染病有检疫传染病、国内未见分布的传染病，还包括登革热、疟疾、流感、禽流感、手足口病、基孔肯雅热、艾滋病等传染病。检疫传染病是指鼠疫、霍乱、黄热病以及国内确定和公布的其他传染病，现在国内已将埃博拉病毒病、新型冠状病毒肺炎纳入检疫传染病管理。国内未见分布传染病是指仅在国外流行或暴发，国内未出现过输入性病例或在国内出现过输入性病例但未造成本土传播的传染病病种，如拉沙热、中东呼吸综合征、寨卡病毒病、裂谷热等。

本章从呼吸道传染病，消化道传染病，蚊媒传染病，经体液、血液、血制品传播的疾病四个方面对口岸重点关注的传染病进行介绍，选择典型传染病分别从病征、传播途径、预防等方面进行阐述。

1.1 呼吸道传染病 Respiratory infectious diseases

1.1.1 新型冠状病毒肺炎① COVID-19

冠状病毒是目前已知 RNA 病毒中基因组最大的病毒，仅感染脊椎动物，其中 7 种能感染人类，包括我们所熟悉的 SARS-CoV（引发重症急性呼吸综合征）和 MERS-CoV（引发中东呼吸综合征）。新型冠状病毒肺炎是指由第 7 种可以感染人的冠状病毒——2019 新型冠状病毒（2019-nCoV）感染引起，以发热、乏力、干咳为主要表现的一种急性呼吸道传染病，人群普遍易感。目前所见传染源主要是新冠病毒感染的患者和无症状感染者，在潜伏期即有传染性，发病后约 5 天内传染性较强。大多数人感染新冠病毒将经历轻中度呼吸道疾病。预防和减缓病毒传播的最好方法是充分了解新冠病

Coronaviruses are the largest known RNA viruses and only infect vertebrates. Seven types of coronaviruses can infect humans, including the familiar SARS-CoV, which causes severe acute respiratory syndrome, and MERS-CoV, which causes Middle East respiratory syndrome. Novel coronavirus pneumonia (COVID-19) is an acute respiratory infectious disease caused by the novel coronavirus 2019 (2019-nCOV), the seventh coronavirus that can infect humans. The main manifestation includes fever, fatigue and dry cough. People are generally susceptible. Currently the main source of infection can be the novel coronavirus infecting patients and asymptomatically infecting people, which has an infectious incubation period, and the infectivity is stronger within about 5 days after COVID-19 onset. Most people infected

① 为方便读者理解，后文"新型冠状病毒"简称为"新冠病毒"，"新型冠状病毒肺炎"简称为"新冠肺炎"。

毒及其引起的疾病和传播方式。

with the COVID-19 virus will experience mild to moderate respiratory illness. The best way to prevent and slow down transmission is to be well informed about the COVID-19 virus, the disease it causes and how it spreads.

1. 临床表现

以发热、乏力、干咳为主要表现。部分患者以嗅觉、味觉减退或丧失等为首发症状，少数患者伴有鼻塞、流涕、咽痛、肌痛和腹泻等症状。患者初期症状通常较轻。一些感染者无任何症状和不适。重症患者多在发病一周后出现呼吸困难和（或）低氧血症，严重者可快速进展为急性呼吸窘迫综合征、脓毒症休克、难以纠正的代谢性酸中毒和出凝血功能障碍及多器官功能衰竭等。

任何人都可能有从轻微到严重的症状。老年人和有严重基础疾病（如心脏病、肺病或糖尿病）的人似乎更有可能患上新冠肺炎的更严重并发症。

1. Clinical features

The most common symptoms of COVID-19 are fever, tiredness, and dry cough. Some patients may first have symptoms of loss of smell and taste. A few patients will have symptoms of nasal congestion, runny nose, sore throat, myalgia, and diarrhea. These symptoms are usually mild at the beginning. Some people become infected but don't develop any symptoms and don't feel unwell. Severe cases usually have dyspnea and/or hypoxemia after one week of onset, and some may rapidly progress to acute respiratory distress syndrome, septic shock, uncorrected metabolic acidosis, hemorrhagic dysfunction, and multiple organ failure.

Anyone can have mild to severe symptoms. Older adults and people who have severe underlying medical conditions like heart or lung disease or diabetes seem to be at higher risk for developing more

新冠肺炎患者可出现各种各样的症状——从轻微症状到严重疾病。接触病毒后 2 ~ 14 天可出现症状。有以下症状的人可能患有新冠肺炎：发热或发冷、咳嗽、呼吸急促或呼吸困难、疲劳、肌肉或身体疼痛、头痛、味觉或嗅觉丧失、咽痛、鼻塞或流涕、恶心或呕吐、腹泻。

2. 潜伏期

基于目前的流行病学调查，潜伏期为 1 ~ 14 天，多为 3 ~ 7 天。

3. 传播途径

经呼吸道飞沫和密切接触传播是主要的传播途径。接触病毒污染的物品也可造成感染。在相对封闭的环境中长时间暴露于高浓度气溶胶情况下存在经气溶胶传播的可能。

4. 病毒变异

随着新冠肺炎疫情的传播，多种新冠病毒变种在全球流行。

serious complications from COVID-19 illness. People with COVID-19 have had a wide range of symptoms—ranging from mild symptoms to severe illness. Symptoms may appear 2 to 14 days after exposure to the virus. People with these symptoms may have COVID-19: fever or chills, cough, shortness of breath or difficulty breathing, fatigue, muscle or body aches, headache, loss of taste and/or smell, sore throat, congestion or runny nose, nausea or vomiting, diarrhea.

2. Incubation period

Based on the current epidemiological investigation, the incubation period is from 1 to 14 days, most are 3 to 7 days.

3. Route of transmission

Transmission of the virus happens mainly through respiratory droplets and close contact. Humans can also be infected by touching objects contaminated by the virus. There is the possibility of aerosol transmission in a relatively closed environment for a long-time exposure to high concentrations of aerosol.

4. Virus variation

Multiple COVID-19 variants are circulating globally as infections spread. In

英国出现了一种携带异常、大量突变的病毒新变种，这一变种似乎比其他变种更容易、更迅速地传播。没有证据表明这种变异会导致更严重的疾病或增加死亡风险。该变异最早于 2020 年 9 月被发现，在伦敦和英格兰东南部非常流行。此后，包括美国和加拿大在内的世界许多国家都发现了这种病毒。

在南非则出现了另一个变种，独立于在英国检测到的变种，该变种最初在 2020 年 10 月初被检测到，与在英国检测到的变种有一些相同的突变。在南非以外，也有这种变种引起的病例。2020 年 12 月在尼日利亚也出现了另一个变种。这些变种似乎比其他变种传播更易、速度更快。没有证据表明这些变种会导致更严重的疾病或增加新冠病毒的传播风险。

the United Kingdom, a new variant has appeared with an unusually large number of mutations. This variant seems to spread more easily and quickly than other variants. There is no evidence that it causes more severe illness or increased risk of death. This variant was first detected in September 2020 and is highly endemic in London and southeast England. Since then, it has been detected in many countries around the world, including the United States and Canada.

In South Africa, another variant appeared independently from the one detected in the UK. The variant was first detected in early October of the same year and has some of the same mutations as the variant detected in the UK. There have also been cases caused by the variant outside South Africa. Another variant appeared in Nigeria in December 2020. These variants seem to spread more easily and quickly than other variants. There is no evidence to indicate these variants are causing more severe illness or increasing the spread of COVID-19.

2021 年 5 月 31 日，世界卫生组织（WHO）宣布了一种新的 COVID-19 变种命名系统。此后，世界卫生组织使用希腊字母来指代在英国、南非和印度等国家首次发现的变异病毒。例如，英国的变体被标记为阿尔法，南非的被标记为贝塔，印度的被标记为德尔塔。世界卫生组织表示，这样标记是为了简化讨论，也有助于消除污名化。

德尔塔变种被称为 B.1.617.2，被认为是迄今为止传播性最强的变种之一，比最初的毒株和在英国首次发现的阿尔法变种更易传播。

2021 年 8 月 30 日，缪变种被世界卫生组织列为"需要留意的变异株"①。世界卫生组织表示，"这种新病毒有可能会逃避疫苗的免疫，有待进一

The World Health Organization(WHO) announced a new naming system for variants of COVID-19 on May 31, 2021. From then on WHO used Greek letters to refer to variants first detected in countries like the UK, South Africa, and India. The UK variant for instance is labelled as Alpha, the South African as Beta, and the Indian as Delta. The WHO said this was to simplify discussions and to help remove some stigma from the names.

Delta, known as B.1.617.2, is believed to be one of the most transmissible variants yet, spreading more easily than both the original strain of the virus and the Alpha variant first identified in Britain.

The Mu variant was newly listed by the World Health Organization as a "variant of interest" on August 30, 2021. The WHO said, "The new virus has the potential to evade immunity from vaccines, pending

---

① 考虑到变异株的传播力和症状等，世界卫生组织将变异株分为"需要关注"和"需要留意"进行监测。目前世界卫生组织将 5 种新冠病毒变异株列为"需要关注的变异株"（Variants of Concern），分别是：最早在英国发现的阿尔法（Alpha）、在南非发现的贝塔（Beta）、在巴西发现的伽马（Gamma）、在印度发现的德尔塔（Delta）和最近在多国发现的奥密克戎（Omicron）。而"需要留意的变异株"（Variants of Interest），级别上低于"需要关注的变异株"。根据世界卫生组织官网显示，缪（Mu）是世界卫生组织列出的第 5 种"需要留意的变异株"，前 4 种分别为：埃塔（Eta）、约塔（Iota）、卡帕（Kappa）和拉姆达（Lambda）。

步研究"。

2021 年 11 月 26 日,世界卫生组织发布声明,将 B. 1. 1. 529 列为"需要关注的变异株",并命名为奥密克戎。世界卫生组织在声明中指出,南非于 11 月 24 日首次将其报告给世界卫生组织,其首个感染该变异株的样本采集时间是 11 月 9 日。① 该变异株包含大量突变。初步研究表明,与其他"需要关注的变异株"相比,该变异株导致人体再次感染病毒的风险增加。

目前已确定的"需要关注的变异株"见表 1-1。

目前已确定的"需要留意的变异株"见表 1-2。

further research. "

On November 26th, 2021, the WHO issued a statement listing B. 1. 1. 529 as a "variant of concern" and named it Omicron. According to a statement by WHO, it was first reported to the WHO by South Africa on the 24th of November and its first sample infected with the mutant strain was collected on the 9th of November. The mutant contains a large number of mutations. Preliminary studies suggest that this variant causes an increased risk of reinfection in humans compared to other " variants of concern".

Currently designated Variants of Concern (VOCs) are shown in Table 1-1.

Currently designated Variants of Interest (VOIs) are shown in Table 1-2.

表 1-1 目前已确定的"需要关注的变异株"

世界卫生组织命名	Pango 谱系②	GISAID 分化枝	Nextstrain 分化枝	监测的其他氨基酸变化③	最早记录的样本	命名日期
阿尔法	B. 1. 1. 7	GRY	20I(V1)	+S: 484K +S: 452R	英国,2020 年 9 月	2020 年 12 月 18 日

---

① 根据世界卫生组织官方数据,2021 年 11 月,除南非外,其他国家也有奥密克戎的样本记录。

② 见世界卫生组织 2021 年 11 月 26 日发表的新冠病毒进化技术咨询小组 (TAG-VE) 声明。

③ 只存在于序列的子集中。

表 1-1 续

世界卫生组织命名	Pango 谱系	GISAID 分化枝	Nextstrain 分化枝	监测的其他氨基酸变化	最早记录的样本	命名日期
贝塔	B.1.351	GH/501Y.V2	20H(V2)	+S: L18F	南非，2020年5月	2020年12月18日
伽马	P.1	GR/501Y.V3	20J(V3)	+S: 681H	巴西，2020年11月	2021年1月11日
德尔塔	B.1.617.2	G/478K.V1	21A, 21I, 21J	+S: 417N +S: 484K	印度，2020年10月	需留意的变异株：2021年4月4日 需关注的变异株：2021年5月11日
奥密克戎	B.1.1.529	GR/484A	21K	—	多个国家，2021年11月	监测中的变异株：2021年11月24日 需关注的变异株：2021年11月26日

Table 1-1 Currently designated Variants of Concern(VOCs)

WHO label	Pango lineage	GISAID clade	Nextstrain clade	Additional amino acid changes monitored	Earliest documented samples	Date of designation
Alpha	B.1.1.7	GRY	20I(V1)	+S: 484K +S: 452R	United Kingdom, Sep-2020	18-Dec-2020
Beta	B.1.351	GH/501Y.V2	20H(V2)	+S: L18F	South Africa, May-2020	18-Dec-2020
Gamma	P.1	GR/501Y.V3	20J(V3)	+S: 681H	Brazil, Nov-2020	11-Jan-2021
Delta	B.1.617.2	G/478K.V1	21A, 21I, 21J	+S: 417N +S: 484K	India, Oct-2020	VOI: 4-Apr-2021 VOC: 11-May-2020
Omicron	B.1.1.529	GR/484A	21K	—	Multiple countries, Nov-2021	VUM: 24-Nov-2021 VOC: 26-Nov-2021

表1-2 目前已确定的"需要留意的变异株"

世界卫生组织命名	Pango 谱系①	GISAID 分化枝	Nextstrain 分化枝	最早记录的样本	命名日期
埃塔	B. 1. 525	G/484K. V3	21D	多个国家，2020年12月	2021年3月17日
约塔	B. 1. 526	GH/253G. V1	21F	美国，2020年11月	2021年3月24日
卡帕	B. 1. 617. 1	G/452R. V3	21B	印度，2020年10月	2021年4月4日
拉姆达	C. 37	GR/452Q. V1	21G	秘鲁，2020年12月	2021年6月14日
缪	B. 1. 621	GH	21H	哥伦比亚，2021年1月	2021年8月30日

Table 1-2 Currently designated Variants of Interest(VOIs)

WHO label	Pango lineage	GISAID clade	Nextstrain clade	Earliest documented samples	Date of designation
Eta	B. 1. 525	G/484K. V3	21D	Multiple countries, Dec-2020	17-Mar-2021
Lota	B. 1. 526	GH/253G. V1	21F	United States of America, Nov-2020	24-Mar-2021
Kappa	B. 1. 617. 1	G/452R. V3	21B	India, Oct-2020	4-Apr-2021
Lambda	C. 37	GR/452Q. V1	21G	Peru, Dec-2020	14-Jun-2021
Mu	B. 1. 621	GH	21H	Colombia, Jan-2021	30-Aug-2021

---

① 见世界卫生组织 2021 年 11 月 26 日发表的新冠病毒进化技术咨询小组（TAG-VE）声明。

5. 疫苗

新冠病毒传染之快、影响之大有目共睹，但限制人员流动并非长久之策。目前应对新冠肺炎有一些特定的疫苗或治疗方法。相比于特效药和抗体治疗，疫苗接种能产生免疫力，是预防性地保护人群并遏制病毒传播既经济且有效的手段。自 2021 年 1 月 2 日起，全球已经有 6 个新冠肺炎疫苗获得正式批准上市，包括美国的辉瑞、德国的拜恩泰科、中国的科兴灭活疫苗等。

目前有若干种疫苗正在使用当中。从每日更新的已接种疫苗剂量数来看，至少有 13 种不同的疫苗（跨越 4 个平台）已投入使用。

2020 年 12 月 31 日，辉瑞和拜恩泰科的复必泰疫苗被纳入世界卫生组织紧急使用列表。2021 年 2 月 16 日，印度血清研究所/Covishield 疫苗和阿斯利康/AZD1222 疫苗被纳入世

5. Vaccine

As we know the novel coronavirus has infected humans and spread quickly and widely, but restrictions to the movement of people cannot be a permanent measure. Currently there are some specific vaccines or treatments for COVID-19. Compared with specific drugs and antibody therapy, vaccination can produce immunity, which is an economical and effective way to protect the population prophylactically and contain the spread of the virus. Six COVID-19 vaccines have been officially approved worldwide since January 2nd, 2021, including the United States' Pfizer vaccine, Germany's BioNTech vaccine, and the inactivated vaccine of China's Sinovac.

There are now several vaccines in use. The number of vaccination doses administered is updated daily. At least 13 different vaccines (across 4 platforms) have been administered.

The Pfizer/BioNTech Comirnaty vaccine was listed for the WHO Emergency Use Listing(EUL) on December 31st, 2020. The SII/Covishield and AstraZeneca/AZD1222 vaccines were listed for EUL on the 16th of February, 2021. The Janssen/

界卫生组织紧急使用列表。2021 年 3 月 12 日，强生公司开发的杨森/Ad26. COV 2. S 疫苗被纳入世界卫生组织紧急使用列表。2021 年 4 月 30 日，莫德纳新冠肺炎疫苗（mRNA 1273）被纳入世界卫生组织紧急使用列表。2021 年 5 月 7 日，国药集团的新冠肺炎疫苗被纳入世界卫生组织紧急使用列表。国药集团疫苗由中国生物技术股份有限公司下属北京生物制品研究所有限责任公司生产。2021 年 6 月 1 日，科兴-克尔来福疫苗被纳入世界卫生组织紧急使用列表。

截至 2022 年 1 月 31 日，世界 61.1% 的人口至少接种了一剂新冠肺炎疫苗，全球已接种 101 亿剂，每天使用 2277 万剂。低收入国家只有 10% 的人至少接种了一剂疫苗。

Ad26. COV 2. S vaccine developed by Johnson & Johnson was listed for EUL on March 12th, 2021. The Moderna COVID-19 vaccine(mRNA 1273) was listed for EUL on April 30th, 2021, and the Sinopharm COVID-19 vaccine was listed for EUL on May 7th, 2021. The Sinopharm vaccine is produced by Beijing Bio-Institute of Biological Products Co. Ltd, subsidiary of China National Biotec Group(CNBG). The Sinovac-CoronaVac was listed for EUL on the 1st of June, 2021.

By January 31, 2022, 61.1% of the world population has received at least one dose of a COVID-19 vaccine. 10.1 billion doses have been administered globally, and 22.77 million are now administered each day. Only 10% of people in low-income countries have received at least one dose.

Words & Expressions

respiratory/'respərətɔːri/ adj. 呼吸的

coronavirus/kə'roʊnəvaɪrəs/ n. 冠状病毒

virus/'vaɪrəs/ n. 病毒

pneumonic/nuː'mɑːnɪk/ adj. 肺炎的

pneumonia/nuː'moʊniə/ n. 肺炎

infected/ɪn'fektɪd/ adj. 受感染的

cross-infection/'krɔːs ɪnfekʃn/ n. 交叉感染

vertebrate/'vɜːrtɪbrət/ n. 脊椎动物；adj. 有脊椎的，脊椎动物的

pandemic/pæn'demɪk/ n. 传染病，流行病

epidemic/ˌepɪ'demɪk/ n.（疾病的）流行，传染

affected/ə'fektɪd/ adj. 感动的，受到影响的，（人或行为）假装的

fatigue/fə'tiːg/ n. 疲劳，厌倦

dizziness/'dɪzinəs/ n. 头昏眼花，头晕

arthralgia/ɑːr'θrældʒə/ n. 关节痛，关节酸痛

dyspnea/dɪsp'niə/ n. 呼吸困难

nausea/'nɔːziə/ n. 作呕，恶心，反胃，极度厌恶

vomit/'vɑmɪt/ v. 呕吐；n. 呕吐物

diarrhea/ˌdaɪə'riə/ n. 腹泻；adj. 腹泻的

stomachache/'stʌmək ˌeɪk/ n. 胃痛，腹痛

hypoxemia/ˌhaɪpɑːk'siːmiə/ n. 血氧不足，血氧过少

epidemiological/ˌepɪˌdiːmiə'lɑːdʒɪkl/ adj. 流行病学的

aerosol/'erəsɑːl/ n. 气溶胶，喷雾剂，悬浮微粒，喷雾器

transmission/ˌtræns'mɪʃn/ n. 传播

clinical/'klɪnɪkl/ adj. 临床的，不带感情的，简陋的

distress/dɪ'stres/ n. 悲伤，痛苦，窘迫；v. 使忧虑，使悲伤，使苦恼

syndrome/'sɪndroʊm/ n. 综合征，综合症状，典型表现

septic/'septɪk/ adj. 脓毒性的，腐败性的

shock/ʃɑːk/ n. 震惊，打击，令人震惊的事，冲击（力）；v. 使震惊，打击

metabolic/ˌmetəˈbɑːlɪk/ adj. 新陈代谢的，变化的

acidosis/ˌæsɪˈdoʊsɪs/ n. 酸液过多症，酸毒症，酸中毒

hemorrhagic/ˌheməˈrædʒɪk/ adj. 出血的，出血性

incubation/ˌɪŋkjuˈbeɪʃn/ n. 孵卵，孵化，［医，生］（传染病的）潜伏期

mutant/ˈmjuːtənt/ n. 突变体，突变异种，变种生物，突变；adj. 突变的，变异的，变异所引起的，经过突变的

stigma/ˈstɪɡmə/ n. 耻辱，污名，烙印，（病的）特征

contagious/kənˈteɪdʒəs/ adj. 感染的，会传染的，富有感染力的

variant/ˈveriənt/ n. 变体

vaccine/vækˈsiːn/ n. 疫苗，菌苗

effective/ɪˈfektɪv/ adj. 有效的

vaccination/ˌvæksɪˈneɪʃn/ n. 疫苗接种

immunity/ɪˈmjuːnəti/ n. 免除，豁免，免疫力

a contagious disease 一场传染性疾病

a more contagious variant 一种更强传染性的变体

novel coronavirus 新型冠状病毒

confirmed case 确诊病例

new confirmed case 新增确诊病例

new suspected case 新增疑似病例

close contact 密切接触者

asymptomatic carrier 无症状感染者

the worst affected/hit 受影响最严重的

mental health 心理健康

running nose 流涕

sore throat 咽痛

muscle pain 肌肉酸痛

shortness of breath 气促

difficulty breathing 呼吸困难

chest tightness　胸闷

chest pain　胸痛

conjunctival congestion　结膜充血

dry cough　干咳

stuffy nose　鼻塞

aerosol transmission　气溶胶传播

clinical signs and symptoms　临床症状

clinically diagnosed case　临床诊断病例

incubation period　潜伏期

mutant strain　变异毒株

effective vaccine　有效疫苗

1.1.2　禽流感　Avian influenza

人感染的禽流感，是由禽流感病毒引起的人类呼吸道传染病。至今发现能直接感染人的禽流感病毒亚型有：H5N1、H7N1、H7N2、H7N3、H7N7、H9N2 和 H7N9 亚型。其中，高致病性 H5N1 亚型和 2013 年 3 月在人体上首次发现的新禽流感 H7N9 亚型尤为引人关注，不仅造成了人类的伤亡，同时重创了家禽养殖业。

Avian influenza that infects humans is a human respiratory infectious disease, caused by avian influenza virus. The already-discovered avian influenza virus subtypes that can directly infect humans are H5N1, H7N1, H7N2, H7N3, H7N7, H9N2 and H7N9. Among them, the highly pathogenic subtype H5N1 and the new avian influenza A subtype (H7N9), which was detected in humans for the first time in March 2013, have attracted particular attention, causing not only human casualties but also severe damage to the poultry industry.

早在 1981 年，美国即有禽流感病毒 H7N7 感染人类引起结膜炎的报道。1997 年中国香港发生 H5N1 型人禽流感导致 6 人死亡，在世界范围内引起了广泛关注。近年来，荷兰、越南、泰国、柬埔寨、印度尼西亚及我国相继出现了人禽流感疫情。该病潜在的风险在于该亚型与人流感病毒存在整合的可能，会导致人与人之间的感染与传播。该病没有特别有效的治疗方法，病死率超过 60%。

Early in 1981, it was reported that humans have conjunctivitis because of infection with the avian influenza virus H7N7 in the United States. The outbreak of H5N1 human avian influenza in Hong Kong, China in 1997, which killed six people, caused widespread concern worldwide. In recent years, there have been human avian influenza outbreaks in the Netherlands, Vietnam, Thailand, Cambodia, Indonesia, and China. The potential risk of this disease lies in the possibility of integration between this subtype and human influenza virus, which will lead to infection and transmission among people. The disease has no particularly effective treatment and the fatality rate is over 60%.

1. 病原体

流感病毒有不同类型。禽流感是由主要感染鸟类和家禽（如鸡或鸭）的流感病毒引起的。由于人类感染禽流感病毒的情况并不常见，因此人体对该病毒的免疫力极低，甚至没有免疫力。

1. Pathogens

There are various types of influenza viruses. Avian influenza is caused by those influenza viruses that mainly affect birds and poultry, such as chickens and ducks. Since the viruses do not commonly infect humans, there is little or no immune protection against them in the human population.

2. 临床表现

人类感染禽流感的病征包括眼部感染（结膜炎）、流感样病征（例如恶心、呕吐、腹泻）或严重的呼吸道感染（例如肺炎）。感染较严重的类型〔如甲型禽流感（H5N1、H5N6、H7N9或H10N8）病毒〕可引致呼吸衰竭、多种器官衰竭，甚至死亡。

3. 传播途径

人类主要通过接触染病的禽鸟（活鸟或死鸟）或其粪便，或接触受污染的环境（例如水产市场和活家禽市场）而感染禽流感病毒。

4. 潜伏期

约7~10天。

5. 预防措施

目前还没有预防人感染禽流感的疫苗。染病的禽鸟（活鸟或死鸟）或其粪便可能带有病毒，因此人们应：

避免接触家禽、雀鸟、动物或其粪便。接触禽鸟或其粪

2. Clinical features

The clinical presentation of avian influenza in humans includes eye infection (conjunctivitis) and flu-like symptoms(e. g. nausea, vomiting and diarrhea) or severe respiratory illness(e. g. pneumonia). Infection of the more virulent forms [e. g. avian influenza A (H5N1, H5N6, H7N9 or H10N8) viruses] can result in respiratory failure, multi-organ failure and even death.

3. Route of transmission

People mainly become infected with avian influenza virus through contact with infected birds and poultry(live or dead) or their droppings or contact with contaminated environments(such as wet markets and live poultry markets).

4. Incubation period

Around 7~10 days.

5. Prevention measures

At present, there is no effective vaccine to prevent avian influenza in humans. Infected birds and poultry (live or dead) or their droppings may carry avian influenza virus. Therefore, members of the public should:

Avoid touching poultry, birds, animals, or their droppings. Wash hands

便后，要立刻用肥皂水或清水彻底洗手。

要彻底煮熟家禽和蛋类食品后进食。

外出旅游时应避免接触禽鸟或其粪便，避免参观家禽市场或农场。旅客从禽流感疫区返回后，若出现流感样症状，应立即求诊，告诉医生最近曾到访的地区，并佩戴外科口罩，以防传染他人。

保持双手清洁，常用肥皂水及清水洗手。

咳嗽或打喷嚏时，用纸巾掩盖口鼻，把用过的纸巾弃置到有害垃圾桶内，然后彻底清洁双手。

如出现流感样症状，应留在家中休息，避免前往拥挤或空气不畅通场所。

保持环境卫生及室内空气流通。

保持均衡饮食、经常运动、充足休息、不要吸烟、避免饮酒，以建立良好的身体抵抗力。

with liquid soap and water immediately and thoroughly after being in contact with birds or poultry or their droppings.

Cook poultry and egg products thoroughly before eating.

Avoid touching birds and poultry or their droppings and visiting poultry markets or farms when travelling. Travelers returning from affected areas with avian influenza outbreaks should consult doctors promptly if they have flu-like symptoms, inform the doctor of their travel history, and wear a surgical mask to prevent the spread of the disease.

Keep hands clean, and wash hands frequently with liquid soap and water.

Cover mouth and/or nose with tissue paper when coughing or sneezing. Dispose of the soiled tissues properly into a lidded trash bin, and then wash hands thoroughly.

Stay at home and avoid going to crowded or poorly ventilated places if having flu-like symptoms.

Maintain environmental hygiene and good indoor ventilation.

Build up a good body immunity by having a balanced diet, regular exercise and adequate rest, do not smoke and avoid alcohol drinking.

Words & Expressions

avian/'eɪvɪən/ adj. 鸟的，鸟类的

influenza/ˌɪnflu'enzə/ n. ［医］流行性感冒，家畜流行性感冒，流感

causative/'kɔːzətɪv/ adj. 成为原因的

poultry/'pəʊltri/ n. 〈集合词〉家禽

virulent/'vɪrələnt/ adj. 剧毒的，致命的，恶毒的，憎恨的

sneeze/'sniːz/ v. 打喷嚏

hygiene/'haɪdʒiːn/ n. 卫生，卫生学，保健法

ventilation/ˌventɪ'leɪʃn/ n. 空气流通，通风设备，通风方法，公开讨论

ventilated/'ventɪleɪtɪd/ adj. 通风的

avian influenza　禽流感

1.1.3　传染性非典型肺炎　Severe acute respiratory syndrome(SARS)

2002 年 11 月，我国广东省部分地区出现了传染性非典型肺炎，两个多月后，该病扩散到我国内地 24 个省、自治区、直辖市。传染性非典型肺炎在全球共波及亚洲、欧洲、美洲等的 32 个国家和地区。截至 2003 年 8 月 7 日，全球累计发病例数 8422 例，死亡 916 例。病死率各年龄层不同，自 0～50%不等，平均病死率达到了 11%。

Severe acute respiratory syndrome (SARS) broke out in parts of Guangdong province in November 2002 and spread to 24 provinces, autonomous regions, and municipalities in the Chinese mainland two months later. It has affected 32 countries and regions in Asia, Europe, and the Americas. As of the 7th of August 2003, 8,422 cases and 916 deaths had been reported globally. The case fatality rate varied by age group, ranging from 0 to 50%, with an average case fatality rate of 11%.

1. 病原体

传染性非典型肺炎是由一种新的冠状病毒（SARS 冠状病毒）引起的一种呼吸系统传染性疾病。该病毒对外界的抵抗力和稳定性强。发病机制尚不清楚，但多数专家认同的观点是，病毒感染诱导的免疫损伤导致了肺部的病变。

2. 临床表现

持续性高热，体温常高于38℃。

干咳，常有流涕、鼻塞、咽痛等上呼吸道卡他症状。

呼吸加速，气促，胸闷，活动后更明显。

3. 传染源

传染性非典型肺炎病人。

4. 传播途径

通过短距离飞沫、接触呼吸道分泌物等途径传播。

5. 易感人群

人群普遍易感。

6. 预防措施

室内经常通风换气，保持

1. Pathogens

Severe acute respiratory syndrome (SARS) is an infectious disease of the respiratory system, caused by a new coronavirus(SARS coronavirus). The virus is highly resistant and stable to outsiders. The pathogenesis is still unclear, but most experts agree that viral-infection-induced immunity leads to lung lesions.

2. Clinical features

Persistent high fever, with body temperature often more than 38℃.

Dry cough, often runny nose, nasal congestion, pharyngeal pain and other upper respiratory tract catarrh symptoms.

Accelerated breathing, shortness of breath and chest tightness, more obvious after activity.

3. Source of infection

SARS patients.

4. Route of transmission

Through short distance droplets, contact with respiratory secretions and other ways of transmission.

5. Susceptible population

The population is generally susceptible.

6. Prevention measures

Keep the room ventilation, maintain

空气流通，勤清洁室内卫生，不给病原微生物滋生机会。

经常到户外活动，呼吸新鲜空气，也可以适当地进行户外运动，锻炼身体，促进身体新陈代谢；多吃新鲜水果蔬菜，补充维生素，提高自身抵抗力，增强体质。

注意均衡饮食和充足休息，减轻精神压力。

保持良好的个人卫生习惯，打喷嚏、咳嗽和清洁鼻腔后要洗手。

尽量避免前往空气流通不畅、人口密集的公共场所。

尽量不要到医院探视病人，必要时戴上口罩，在疾病流行期间尽量不要去人多的地方，外出最好戴上口罩，以防交叉感染。

air circulation, keep indoor sanitation and do not give the opportunities of pathogenic microorganisms to breed.

Go outdoors often, breathe fresh air, practice outdoor activities, exercise, and promote the body metabolism system; eat some fresh fruits and vegetables, take supplements and vitamins, improve body resistance and enhance physical fitness.

Pay attention to a well-balanced diet and get adequate rest to relieve mental stress.

Maintain good personal hygiene habits and wash hands after sneezing, coughing and cleaning nasal cavities.

Try to avoid going to public places with poor air circulation and dense population.

Try not to visit patients in hospitals, wear masks when necessary, and try not to go to crowded places during the epidemic. It is best to wear masks when going out to prevent cross-infection.

Words & Expressions

SARS/saːz/ n. 传染性非典型肺炎（severe acute respiratory syndromes）

severe/sɪ'vɪr/ adj. 严重的

acute/ə'kjuːt/ adj. 急性的

syndrome/'sɪndroʊm/ n. 综合征，综合症状，典型表现

pathogen/'pæθədʒən/ n. 病菌，病原体

catarrh/kə'tɑːr/ n. ［医］卡他，黏膜炎

metabolism/mə'tæbəlɪzəm/ n. 新陈代谢，代谢作用

1.1.4 鼠疫 Plague

鼠疫是一种烈性检疫传染病，人类可以通过被鼠疫杆菌感染的跳蚤叮咬、与受鼠疫杆菌污染的物品直接接触或吸入含鼠疫杆菌的飞沫感染。1911年年初，中国黑龙江哈尔滨出现首例肺鼠疫病例，同年12月，鼠疫进入暴发期。1912年1月8日，因鼠疫死亡人数达到150人。此后，鼠疫在非洲、美洲和亚洲的许多国家流行。2003年，9个国家共报告了2118例病例和182人死亡，其中98.7%的病例和98.9%的死亡是由非洲报告的。鼠疫的分

Plague is a kind of fulminating quarantinable infectious disease. Humans can be infected by the bites of infected fleas, by direct contact with infected materials or by inhalation of droplets containing bacteria. In early 1911, the first pneumonic plague appeared in Harbin, Heilongjiang, China. In December of the same year, the plague outbreak began. On January 8th, 1912, the death toll reached 150. Since then, plagues have become endemic in many countries in Africa, the Americas, and Asia. In 2003, a total of 2,118 cases and 182 deaths were reported from nine countries, of which 98.7% of

布与其自然疫源地的地理分布相一致。

马达加斯加曾于 2017 年 8 月暴发鼠疫疫情。世界卫生组织发布了橙色 2 级预警，认定南非、莫桑比克、坦桑尼亚、毛里求斯、科摩罗、塞舌尔、留尼汪岛、埃塞俄比亚和肯尼亚 9 个国家为鼠疫暴发高风险国家。本病发病急，病情重，以往病死率极高，几乎无幸存者，近年由于抗生素（链霉素、四环素、氯霉素）的及时应用，病死率降至 5%~10%。

1. 病原体和临床表现

该烈性传染病由鼠疫杆菌引起，鼠疫杆菌多自皮肤侵入人体淋巴结，引起出血性坏死性炎症，另外也可从呼吸道侵入肺组织。肺部病变以充血、水肿、出血为主，病菌释放毒素进入血液循环引起败血症，全身各器官均可有出血、坏死改变。

cases and 98.9% of deaths were reported from Africa. The distribution of plagues corresponds to the geographical distribution of its natural epidemic focus.

An outbreak of a plague began in Madagascar in August 2017. The World Health Organization has issued an Orange Level 2 Warning and confirmed the following nine countries—South Africa, Mozambique, Tanzania, Mauritius, Comoros, Seychelles, Reunion Island, Ethiopia, and Kenya as high-risk countries of plague outbreaks. The onset of this disease is acute and severe, accompanied by high fatality rate and almost no survivors. In recent years, due to the timely application of antibiotics（streptomycin, tetracycline, chloramphenicol）, the case fatality rate has been declined to 5% to 10%.

1. Pathogens and clinical features

The fierce infectious disease is caused by the plague bacillus, which invades the human lymph nodes through the skin, causing hemorrhagic necrotizing inflammation. It can also invade lung tissue from the respiratory tract additionally. Lung lesions are manifested mainly by hyperemia, oedema, hemorrhage, and the pathogen releases a toxin into the blood circulation, causing septicemia, and all organs of the whole body can have hemorrhage, necrotic change.

2. 潜伏期

鼠疫的潜伏期较短，一般为1~6天，多为2~3天，个别病例达到8~9天。

3. 传染源

主要是鼠类及鼠疫病人。

4. 传播途径

经鼠蚤叮咬传播。

经直接接触传播。通过捕猎、宰杀、剥皮及食肉等方式直接接触染疫动物而感染。食用未煮熟的鼠疫病死动物（如旱獭、兔、藏系绵羊等）可发生肠鼠疫。

经飞沫传播。肺鼠疫患者或动物呼吸道分泌物中含有大量鼠疫杆菌，形成细菌微粒及气溶胶，造成肺鼠疫传播。

实验室感染。由于防护不严、操作不当和实验室事故造成感染。

2. Incubation period

Plague has a short incubation period. The incubation period of plague is usually from 1 to 6 days, mostly 2 to 3 days, even up to 8 to 9 days in rare cases.

3. Source of infection

Mainly rats and plague patients.

4. Route of transmission

Transmitted by rats and flea bites.

Transmitted by direct contact. The infection is caused by direct contact with infected animals through hunting, slaughtering, flaying, and eating. Intestinal plague may occur by eating uncooked dead animals (such as marmots, rabbits, Tibetan sheep, etc.).

Transmitted by droplet. Pneumonic plague patients or animal's respiratory secretions contain a large number of plague bacilli, which form bacterial particles and aerosols, causing the spread of pneumonic plague.

Laboratory infection. Infection occurs due to inadequate protection, improper operation, and laboratory accidents.

5. 易感人群

人群普遍易感。到过鼠疫自然疫源地或接触过鼠疫疫区内的疫源动物、动物制品及鼠疫病人的人感染风险更高。

6. 预防措施

尽量减少赴疫情流行地区旅行。如果需要赴疫情流行地区旅行，应采取佩戴口罩、勤洗手等个人防护措施，避免接触鼠等啮齿和病/死动物。可使用针对蚊虫的驱虫产品，避免跳蚤叮咬。

避免与有发热、咳嗽、淋巴结肿大、头痛、腹泻等症状的病人接触，不参加人群聚集活动，不参加当地人的葬礼。

如怀疑已接触鼠疫患者，或在疫情发生地被跳蚤叮咬，应立即咨询医生获取帮助。

如果出现发热、咳嗽、淋巴结肿大、头痛、腹泻等症状，建议取消或推迟回国行程，及时就医并告知当地使领馆工作

5. Susceptible population

The population is generally susceptible. People who have been to plague natural foci or contact with plague source animals, animal products and plague patients in plague epidemic areas are at higher risk of infection.

6. Prevention measures

Please minimize travel to the epidemic areas. If you need to travel to epidemic areas, you should take personal protective measures such as wearing masks, washing your hands to avoid contact with rodents, sick or dead animals, and using insect repellents to avoid flea bites.

Avoid contact with patients who have symptoms such as fever, cough, swollen lymph nodes, headache and diarrhea. Do not participate in crowd gatherings or attend local funerals.

You should seek medical help immediately if you were suspected to have been exposed to plague patients or bitten by fleas in the epidemic region.

If you have symptoms such as fever, cough, swollen lymph nodes, headache, diarrhea, etc., it is recommended to cancel or postpone the trip back to China, seek

人员。

归国途中如出现上述症状，应向乘务人员主动申报，并配合乘务人员工作。

从疫情发生地归国入境时，如出现上述症状，应向海关主动申报并告知旅行史和接触史，配合海关人员工作。

入境后，应当密切关注身体状况，如出现上述症状，应当立即就医并告知旅行史和接触史，同时通知当地检疫机构。

medical advice and inform the staff of the local embassy and consulate.

If any of these symptoms occur on the way back to your country, you should report to the crew and cooperate with them.

If the above-mentioned symptoms appear, you should report proactively to the customs and inform about your travel records and contact history, and cooperate with the customs officials when returning from the place where the outbreak occurred.

After you entered the country, you should pay close attention to your physical condition. If the above symptoms occur, you should seek medical treatment immediately and inform about your travel records and contact history, and report to the local quarantine authorities.

Words & Expressions

plague/pleɪg/ n. 传染病，鼠疫

fulminate/'fʊlmɪneɪt/ v. 强烈批评

inhalation/ˌɪnhə'leɪʃn/ n. 吸入，吸入剂，吸入物

antibiotic/ˌæntibaɪ'ɑːtɪk/ n. （用作复数）抗生素

lesion/'liːʒn/ n. 损害，身体器官组织的损伤，感染性的皮肤

hemorrhage/'hemərɪdʒ/ n. 出血（尤指大出血）

hyperemia/ˌhaɪpə'riːmɪə/ n. 充血

oedema/ɪ'diːmə/ n. 水肿，瘤腺体

septicemia/ˌseptɪˈsiːmɪə/ n. 败血病

necrotic/neˈkrɑːtɪk/ adj. 坏死的，坏疽的，骨疽的

susceptible/səˈseptəbl/ adj. 易受影响的，易受感染的，善感的，可以接受的

cholera plague　霍乱疫情

1. 1. 5　流感　Influenza

"流感"，全称"流行性感冒"，是由流感病毒引起的一类以发热为主的急性呼吸道传染病。流感病毒分为甲、乙、丙、丁四型，其中甲型流感病毒变异性强，而且传染性强，传播迅速，易引起流感流行或大流行；乙型流感病毒可引起流感局部暴发，每年和甲型流感病毒共同循环引起季节性流行；丙型流感病毒一般呈散发感染；丁型主要感染牛，尚未发现人类感染。

人类历史上曾多次发生流感世界大流行，主要有1918年发生的"西班牙流感"，1957年发生的"亚洲流感"和2009年发生的甲型H1N1流感。由

"The flu" full name "influenza", is a class of acute respiratory infectious disease with fever caused by influenza virus. Influenza virus is divided into A, B, C and D types. Among them, the influenza A virus is highly variable and infectious, which spreads so quickly that it can easily cause influenza or pandemic. Influenza B virus can cause local outbreaks of influenza and circulate with influenza A virus every year to cause seasonal epidemics. Influenza C virus infection is generally sporadic. Influenza D mainly infects cattle and has not been found in humans yet.

There have been many worldwide influenza pandemics in human history, including the "Spanish flu" in 1918, the "Asian flu" in 1957, and the H1N1 influenza in 2009. Influenza pandemic caused serious losses to human health and

于传染性强、并发症严重、死亡率高，流感大流行给人类健康和社会经济造成了严重损失。1918 年的西班牙流感大流行席卷全球，感染人数超过 6 亿，夺去了 2000 多万人的生命。

流感一年四季都可流行，但多发于冬季，原因是冬季寒冷，人体抵抗力减弱，同时冬季室内活动较多，空气流通不畅，易导致病毒传播。

1. 临床表现

其病症为起病急，发热，体温可高达 39℃～40℃，伴畏寒、寒战、头痛、全身酸痛、极度乏力、食欲减退等全身症状，且常有眼睛干涩、喉咙干燥、咽痛、咳嗽。部分病人有喷嚏、流涕、鼻塞、结膜轻度充血。有时可见胃肠道症状，如恶心、呕吐、腹泻等。

流感不同于预后良好的普通感冒，病程一般要十几天，而且易引发严重的并发症，如

social economy due to its high infectivity, serious complications, and high mortality. The 1918 Spanish flu pandemic swept the world, infecting more than 600 million people and killing more than 20 million.

Influenza can be prevalent throughout the year, but more in winter. The reason is that cold winter makes people's immunity weakened. At the same time indoor activities are more popular in winter, and poor air circulation may easily lead to the spread of the virus.

1. Clinical features

Influenza is characterized by sudden occurrence. Patients have fever with systemic symptoms such as chills, headache, body ache, weakness, poor appetite, often with dry eyes, dry throat, mild pharyngeal pain, cough, and body temperature can be as high as 39℃ to 40℃. Some patients may have sneeze, runny nose, nasal congestion, and mild conjunctiva congestion. Sometimes patients have gastrointestinal symptoms such as nausea, vomiting, diarrhea, etc.

Influenza is different from the common cold with good prognosis. The course of illness generally takes more than ten days,

肺炎、急性呼吸窘迫综合征、喉炎、心肌炎等，后果严重。

2. 传播途径

主要通过空气飞沫传播。

3. 预防措施

自我保护。保持个人卫生，勤洗手。注意锻炼身体，增强对各种疾病的抵抗力。在流感的高发期，注意室内通风，保持清洁，尽量少到人群密集的地方。不接触病禽和病畜。

疫苗接种。对高危人群、易感人群，接种流感疫苗是预防流感的有效方法。由于流感病毒变异非常活跃，这种特异性保护作用只能维持一年。正在患发热性疾病的病人、急性感染期和慢性病活动期的病人应推迟接种。对鸡蛋过敏者不能接种。

服用预防药物。必要时，在医生的指导下，可服用抗流感病毒的针对性药物，如金刚

and it is easy to cause serious complications, such as pneumonia, asthma, laryngitis, myocarditis and so on, with serious consequences.

2. Route of Transmission

Mainly transmitted through air droplets.

3. Prevention measures

Self-protection. Maintain personal hygiene and wash hands frequently. Pay attention to physical exercise, and strengthen the immunity to various diseases. In the peak season of influenza, pay attention to indoor ventilation, keep clean and away from crowded places, and avoid contact with sick poultry and livestock.

Vaccination. Influenza vaccination is an effective way to prevent influenza among high-risk and susceptible groups. The flu virus mutates so actively that this specific protection can only last for one year. Patients who are suffering from febrile illness, acute infection and chronic disease should postpone vaccination. People allergic to eggs cannot get vaccinated.

Take preventive medicine. When necessary, under the guidance of doctors, people can take targeted drugs against influenza virus, such as amantadine,

烷胺、金刚乙胺，有条件的可选用达菲，也可选用野菊花、板蓝根等中药进行预防。

rimantadine. Tamiflu can be used if conditions are met. People can also choose wild chrysanthemum, radix isatidis and other traditional Chinese medicine for prevention.

Words & Expressions

manifestation/ˌmænɪfeˈsteɪʃn/ n. 临床表现，表示，显示

asthma/ˈæzmə/ n. 气喘，哮喘

laryngitis/ˌlærɪnˈdʒaɪtɪs/ n. 喉炎

myocarditis/ˌmaɪokɑrˈdaɪtɪs/ n. 心肌炎

chrysanthemum/krɪˈsænθəməm/ n. 菊花，菊属

1.1.6 肺炭疽 Pulmonary anthrax

肺炭疽是一种由炭疽杆菌引发的急性呼吸道传染病。首发症状与普通感冒相似，但随后快速进展为严重的呼吸困难和休克。全球均有散发病例。多见于亚洲、非洲和南美洲。

Pulmonary anthrax is a kind of acute respiratory contagious disease caused by bacillus anthracis. The initial symptoms are similar to the common cold but can quickly develop to severe breathing difficulties and shock. There are sporadic cases worldwide, most common in Asia, Africa and South America.

1. 病原体和临床表现

大多为原发性，由吸入炭疽杆菌所致，也可继发皮肤感

1. Pathogens and clinical features

The disease is mostly primary and caused by inhalation of bacillus anthracis,

染。起病急，但一般先有 2～4 天感冒样症状，且在缓解后再突然起病。临床表现为寒战、高热、气急、呼吸困难、喘鸣、发绀、血样痰、胸痛，有时在颈下、胸部出现皮下水肿，病情多危重，常并发败血症和感染性休克，偶可继发脑膜炎。如不及时抢救，24～48 小时可因呼吸、循环衰竭死亡。

2. 潜伏期

潜伏期一般 1～5 天，短者 12 小时也可发病，长者则可能于两周后发病。

3. 传播途径

肺炭疽主要通过呼吸道吸入带有炭疽杆菌芽孢的粉尘或气溶胶引起，也可继发于皮肤炭疽。夏秋季节多发。

and skin infections may be followed. Symptoms prior to the onset of the final hyperacute phase are nonspecific, like common flu for 2 to 4 days. The mild initial phase of nonspecific symptoms is followed by sudden development of dyspnea, disorientation with coma, and death. The clinical manifestations include chilly, high-grade fever, cyanosis, bloody sputum, and chest pain. Subcutaneous edema on neck or chest may occur. Complications like septicemia, shock and rarely meningitis can be fatal. Death caused by respiratory failure or circulatory failure may occur within 24 to 48 hours if rescue measures fail.

2. Incubation preiod

The incubation period ranges between 1 and 5 days. The symptoms can appear quickly in 12 hours or over 2 weeks after exposure.

3. Route of transmission

Pulmonary anthrax is mainly caused by inhalation of dust or aerosols containing anthrax bacillus spores through the respiratory tract and can also be secondary to cutaneous anthrax infection. Most happen in summer and autumn.

4. 预防措施

旅行前，请向医生咨询目的地该病流行情况。

旅行时，注意保持所在场所通风，注意个人卫生。去污、消毒和正确处理感染或污染了的物品是预防国际传播最重要的手段。抗生素预防仅推荐用于已知或高度怀疑因蓄意释放而被暴露于大剂量含炭疽杆菌芽孢的气溶胶。①

旅行回国入境时或入境后，如出现相关症状，应主动向海关报告，并尽早到医院治疗，主动告知医生近期旅行情况。

4. Prevention measures

Consult a doctor about the epidemic situation of the destination before travel.

While travel, keep the environment ventilated and clean, and maintain good hygiene habits. Disinfection, decontamination, correct disposal of contaminated materials are very important in preventing transmission of anthrax. Prolonged antibiotic prophylaxis is only a recommendation for persons known to have been or strongly suspected of having been exposed to very substantial doses of aerosolized spores in a deliberate release scenario.

After travel, if related symptoms of pulmonary anthrax develop, report to customs proactively, see a doctor and inform him/her about your recent patient contact history, travel history and so on.

Words & Expressions

anthrax/'ænθræks/ n. ［医］炭疽（病），炭疽脓疱

bacillus/bə'sɪləs/ n. 杆菌，芽孢杆菌属

spore/spɔːr/ n. （细菌、苔藓、蕨类植物）孢子

cyanosis/ˌsaɪə'noʊsɪs/ n. 发绀，苍白病，黄萎病

subcutaneous/ˌsʌbkju'teɪnɪəs/ adj. 皮下的

cutaneous/kju'teɪnɪəs/ adj. 皮肤的，影响皮肤的

① 少数国家批准疫苗用于特定年龄人群有暴露高风险时。

edema/ɪ'diːmə/ n. 水肿，浮肿，瘤腺体

disorientation/dɪsˌɔːriən'teɪʃn/ n. 方向障碍，迷惑

prolonged/prə'lɔːŋd/ adj. 持续很久的，延长的，拖延的

prophylaxis/ˌproʊfə'læksɪs/ n. 预防

scenario/sə'nærioʊ/ n. 设想，可能发生的情况

1.1.7 军团菌病 Legionnaires disease

军团菌病是由军团菌属细菌所致的临床综合征，是以肺炎为主的全身性疾病。本病可散发，亦可暴发流行。军团菌病呈世界性分布。流行季节为7~9月，散发病例四季皆有。

Legionnaires disease is a clinical syndrome caused by legionella bacteria, which is mainly a systemic disease of pneumonia. Legionnaires disease can cause emanation or outbreak. Legionnaires disease is ubiquitous worldwide. The disease is endemic with seasonal distribution from July to September. Emanation cases can occur all over the year.

1. 临床表现

起病缓慢，但也可经2~10天潜伏期而急骤发病。主要表现为发热、咳嗽，伴胸痛、肌痛及乏力。

1. Clinical features

Legionnaires disease typically presents with pneumonia. Symptom onset occurs in 2 to 10 days after exposure, which is characterized by fever, cough, myalgia, chest aches and atony.

2. 传播途径

军团菌病可通过吸入含有细菌的水溶性气溶胶传播。军团菌可在温暖潮湿环境生长。

2. Route of transmission

Transmission occurs by inhalation of water aerosol containing the bacteria. The bacterium grows in warm fresh-water

该病不会人传人。

environments. Person-to-person transmission does not occur with either legionnaires disease.

3. 预防措施

旅行前，请向医生了解目的地该病流行情况。

旅行时要留意居留场所的卫生状况，房间要多通风，不饮生水，所住酒店有疫情发生时可佩戴口罩加强个人防护。

旅行后近期凡有发热、大汗、咳嗽，咳白、黏痰，伴胸痛、肌痛及乏力等相关病征，应尽早到医院诊治，主动告知最近旅行史。

3. Prevention measures

Consult doctors about the epidemic situation of the destination before travel.

During the journey, maintain healthy habits to avoid consumption of contaminated water, and live in rooms with good ventilation. Reinforce protection by using mask if epidemic occurs in the hotel you check in.

See a doctor for diagnosis and treatment as early as possible and tell him/her the recent travel history if there is a sudden onset of relevant symptoms after travel.

Words & Expressions

genus/ˈdʒiːnəs/ n.（动植物的）属，类，种，型

legionnaire/ˌliːdʒəˈner/ n. 美国退伍军人协会会员，军团的士兵

legionella/ˌliːdʒəˈnelə/ n. ［医］（复 legionellae）军团杆菌，军团杆菌属

ubiquitous/juːˈbɪkwɪtəs/ adj. 无所不在的，普遍存在的

emanation/ˌeməˈneɪʃn/ n. 发射，散发，发射物，（由衰变产生的）射气

atony/ˈætəni/ n.（尤指收缩器官的）张力缺乏，迟缓，无重音，无重读

1.1.8 中东呼吸综合征 Middle East respiratory syndrome

中东呼吸综合征（MERS）是由 MERS 冠状病毒感染引起的急性严重呼吸道疾病。2012年首次出现在沙特，此后，约旦、卡塔尔、阿联酋、突尼斯乃至法国、德国、英国、美国等先后发现该病确诊病例。截至 2022 年 2 月，全球共报告 2585 例实验室确诊病例，890 例死亡，病死率 34.4%；其中 2184 例报告自沙特阿拉伯。还未有针对性治疗此病的方法，主要为支持性治疗。

1. 病原体

冠状病毒可分为很多种类，其中包括可能导致轻微疾病如普通感冒的病毒，亦可引致严重的疾病，如传染性非典型肺炎（SARS）。冠状病毒有三种主要类别，包括：alpha（α）、beta（β）和 gamma（γ）。MERS 冠状病毒属于 β 类别，

Middle East respiratory syndrome (MERS) is an acute, severe respiratory disease caused by novel coronavirus MERS-CoV infection. The disease was first reported in Saudi Arabia in 2012. Since then, confirmed cases have been found in Jordan, Qatar, the United Arab Emirates, Tunisia, even in France, Germany, the United Kingdom, and the United States. As of February 2022, a total of 2,585 laboratory-confirmed cases and 890 deaths were reported worldwide, with a case fatality rate of 34.4%. Of these, 2,184 cases were reported from Saudi Arabia. There is no specific treatment for the disease, and it is mainly supportive care.

1. Pathogens

Coronaviruses are a large family of viruses which include viruses that may cause mild illness like common cold as well as severe illness like severe acute respiratory syndrome (SARS) in humans. There are 3 main subgroups of coronaviruses: alpha(α), beta(β) and gamma(γ). MERS-CoV is a beta coronavirus which has not been

以往从未在人类中发现，亦跟曾在人类或动物上所发现的冠状病毒（包括引致 SARS 的冠状病毒）不同。

identified in humans before and is different from any coronaviruses (including SARS-coronavirus) that have been found in humans or animals.

2. 临床表现

患者可出现急性严重呼吸系统疾病，症状包括发烧、咳嗽、呼吸急促和困难。多数患者患有肺炎或出现肾脏衰竭等严重并发症。很多病人还有肠胃方面的症状，如腹泻和恶心/呕吐。免疫力较弱的患者，可出现非典型病症。

2. Clinical features

Infected persons may present with acute serious respiratory illness with symptoms including fever, cough, shortness of breath and breathing difficulties. Most patients developed severe complications such as pneumonia and kidney failure. Many also had gastrointestinal symptoms including diarrhea and nausea/vomiting. For those people with immune deficiencies, the disease may have atypical presentation.

3. 传播途径

可通过接触动物（尤其是骆驼）、环境或确诊病人（例如在医院内）而受感染。一般冠状病毒的传播途径，与其他呼吸道感染如流感相似。此外，一些科学研究证实骆驼为 MERS 冠状病毒的主要来源。

3. Route of transmission

People may be infected upon exposure to animals(especially camel), environment or other confirmed patients(such as in a hospital setting). Coronaviruses typically spread like other respiratory infections such as influenza. Besides, scientific studies support those camels served as the primary source of MERS-CoV.

4. 潜伏期

2~14 天。

4. Incubation period

2 to 14 days.

5. 预防措施

如出现呼吸道感染症状时，

5. Prevention measures

Wear surgical mask and seek medical advice promptly if respiratory symptoms

应佩戴外科口罩，并尽快求诊。

注意保持个人卫生和环境卫生，防止疾病传播。

打喷嚏或咳嗽时应用纸巾掩着口鼻，并将污染的纸巾妥善弃置于有盖垃圾箱内。

保持均衡饮食、规律运动、充足休息，不吸烟和避免饮酒，以建立良好身体抵抗力。

虽然冠状病毒可能会在环境中存活一段时间，但一般清洁剂都能轻易地消灭此病毒。要保持家居清洁，避免前往人多拥挤、空气欠流通的地方，保持空气流通。

避免到访农场、农庄及有骆驼的集市。

旅程中避免接触骆驼（包括骑骆驼或涉及接触骆驼的活动）、雀鸟、家禽或病人。

一旦到访农场、农庄或有骆驼的集市，接触动物前后均应经常洗手。

develop.

Pay attention to personal and environmental hygiene to prevent the spread of disease.

Cover nose and mouth with tissue paper while sneezing or coughing and dispose of soiled tissue paper in a lidded rubbish bin.

Build up good body immunity by having a balanced diet, regular exercise, and adequate rest, do not smoke and avoid alcohol consumption.

Though coronaviruses may survive for some time in the environment, they are easily destroyed by most detergents and cleaning agents. It is important to keep our home clean, avoid visiting crowded places with poor ventilation and maintain good ventilation.

Avoid going to farms, barns and markets with camels.

Avoid contact with camels (including riding camels or participating in any activity involving contact with camels), birds, poultry, or sick people during travel.

Wash hands regularly before and after touching animals in case of visits to farms, barns or markets with camels.

避免近距离接触病人，特别是有急性呼吸道感染症状的病人，以及避免到中东呼吸综合征病人入住的医护环境。

应注意食物安全和卫生，避免进食或饮用生或未熟透的动物产品，包括奶和肉类，或食用可能被动物分泌物、排泄物（例如尿液）或产品污染的食物，除非已经煮熟、洗净或妥为去皮。

如佩戴外科口罩感到不适应，应尽快求医，告知医生近期的旅行史。

Avoid close contact with sick people, especially with those suffering from acute respiratory infections, and avoid visit to healthcare settings with MERS patients.

Adhere to food safety and hygiene rules such as avoiding consuming raw or undercooked animal products, including milk and meat, or foods which may be contaminated by animal secretions, excretions (such as urine) or products, unless they have been properly cooked, washed or peeled.

If feeling unwell, put on a surgical mask, seek medical attention immediately and inform the doctor of your recent travel history.

Words & Expressions

gastrointestinal/ˌɡæstrouɪnˈtestɪnl/ adj. 胃与肠的

intestinal/ɪnˈtestɪnl/ adj. 肠的，肠壁，肠道细菌

deficiency/dɪˈfɪʃənsi/ n. 缺乏，不足，缺陷，瑕疵，赤字

detergent/dɪˈtɜːrdʒənt/ n. 洗涤剂，去污剂；adj. 使清洁的，（与）清洁添加剂（有关）的

barn/bɑːrn/ n. 畜棚，谷仓，空荡荡的大建筑，（停放汽车、火车等的）大车库

1.2 消化道传染病 Infectious diseases of the digestive tract

1.2.1 霍乱 Cholera

在 1817 年至今的 200 多年间，霍乱在亚、非、欧、美各洲曾先后发生过 7 次世界性大流行，无一祸及中国。始于 1961 年的第七次霍乱大流行由埃尔托生物型引发，至今已 60 余年，其持续时间之长，波及范之广，超过以前的历次流行。进入 20 世纪 90 年代，情况更为严峻，随着霍乱入侵拉丁美洲，1991 年美洲报告了近 40 万霍乱病例，同年全球病例达到 60 万，是第七次霍乱大流行病例报告最多的一年。四环素、诺氟沙星可减轻腹泻，目前流行的埃尔托生物型霍乱的病死率已在 1% 之下，但如不治疗，病死率大于 50%。

1. 病原体

霍乱是由霍乱弧菌引起的疾病。霍乱弧菌为革兰氏阴性

Cholera is an international quarantinable infectious disease. Cholera occurred seven times in Asia, Africa, Europe, and the Americas during the 200 years since 1817, none of which hit China. The seventh pandemic, which began in 1961 and was caused by the El tobiome, has lasted longer and more widely than any previous pandemic for more than 60 years. In the 1990s, the situation became even more serious as cholera invaded Latin America with nearly 400,000 cases in the Americas in 1991. 600,000 cases were reported globally in the same year, the highest number of cases in the seventh cholera pandemic. Tetracycline and norfloxacin can alleviate diarrhea. The mortality rate of the current epidemic Elto biotype disorder is less than 1%, but more than 50% without treatment.

1. Pathogens

Cholera is caused by the bacterium Vibrio cholerae. Vibrio cholerae is Gram

菌，对干燥、日光、热、酸及一般消毒剂均敏感。霍乱弧菌产生致病性的是内毒素及外毒素。

2. 临床表现

正常胃酸可杀死霍乱弧菌，当胃酸分泌暂时低下或入侵病菌数量增多时，未被胃酸杀死的弧菌进入小肠，在碱性肠液内迅速繁殖，并产生大量强烈的外毒素。这种外毒素作用于小肠黏膜，引起肠液的大量分泌，超过肠管再吸收的能力，在临床上出现剧烈泻吐，严重脱水，致使血浆容量明显减少，体内盐分缺乏，血液浓缩，出现周围循环衰竭。由于剧烈泻吐、电解质丢失、缺钾缺钠、肌肉痉挛、酸中毒等，该病甚至引发休克及急性肾衰竭。

3. 潜伏期

潜伏期为 1~3 天，通常为

negative and sensitive to dryness, sunlight, heat, acid, and general disinfectants. The pathogenicity of Vibrio cholerae is endotoxin and exotoxin.

2. Clinical features

Normal gastric acid can kill Vibrio cholerae. When the gastric acid is temporarily low or the number of invading bacteria increases, the Vibrio that has not been killed by gastric acid enters the small intestine, propagates rapidly in alkaline intestinal juice, and produces a large number of strong exotoxins. The effect of this exotoxin on the small intestinal mucosa causes a large amount of secretion of intestinal fluid, which exceeds the ability of intestinal re-absorption. It may have the clinic symptoms of severe diarrhea and vomiting, severe dehydration, resulting in a significant reduction of plasma volume, lack of salt in body, blood concentration, and peripheral circulation failure. Due to severe diarrhea and vomiting, electrolyte loss, lack of potassium and sodium, muscle spasm, acidosis, it even causes shock and acute renal failure.

3. Incubation period

The incubation period is 1 to 3 days

突然发病。

4. 传染源

病人及带菌者是主要的传染源。

5. 传播途径

通过被霍乱弧菌污染的水或食物传播。病人及带菌者的粪便污染水源或食物后引起传播，其中水源污染在霍乱传播中最为主要。

6. 易感人群

人群普遍易感，隐性感染多，显性感染少。感染后获得免疫，但持续时间短，会再次感染。

7. 预防措施

健康教育。要大力加强以预防肠道传染病为重点的宣传教育，提倡喝开水，不吃生的/半生的食物，生吃瓜果要洗净，饭前要洗手，养成良好的卫生习惯。

免疫接种。目前尚无理想

and the onset of cholera usually occurs abruptly.

4. Source of infection

Patients and carriers are the main source of infection.

5. Route of transmission

It is transmitted by water or food polluted by Vibrio cholerae. The transmission of cholera is caused by contaminated feces and feces of patients and carriers, mainly by water pollution.

6. Susceptible population

The population is generally susceptible, more with inapparent infection and less with apparent infection. Humans become immune after infection, but it lasts for a short time and then humans can be infected again.

7. Prevention measures

Health education. We should vigorously strengthen the publicity and education focusing on the prevention of intestinal infectious diseases. Drink boiled water, do not eat raw/half-raw food, and wash raw fruits and melons before eating. Maintain good health habits, and wash hands before meals.

Immunization. There is no ideal cholera vaccine with good protection effect

的、保护效果较好和保护持续时间较长的霍乱菌苗，因此不提倡使用过去沿用的霍乱疫苗用于霍乱的预防。

and long protection duration at present, so the cholera vaccine used in the past is not recommended for cholera prevention.

加强饮用水卫生。要加快城乡自来水建设。保护水源，改善饮用水条件，在一时达不到要求的地区，实行饮水消毒。

Strengthen drinking water sanitation management. Accelerate the construction of urban and rural tap water. It is necessary to protect source of water, improve conditions of drinking water and disinfect drinking water in areas that cannot meet the requirements for the time being.

抓好饮食卫生。严格执行《中华人民共和国食品卫生法》，特别要加强对饮食行业（包括餐厅、个体饮食店、小摊档等）、农贸集市、集体食堂等的卫生管理。

Pay attention to food hygiene. Strictly implement Food Hygiene Law of the People's Republic of China, and especially strengthen the hygiene management of catering industry (including restaurants, individual catering stores, stalls, etc.), farmers' markets and canteens.

Words & Expressions

cholera/ˈkɑːlərə/ n. 霍乱

vibrio/ˈvɪbrɪˌo/ n. 弧菌（一种 S 形霍乱菌），[医] 弧菌属

tetracycline/ˌtetrəˈsaɪklɪn/ n. 四环素

norfloxacin/nɔrflɒkˈseɪsɪn/ n. [化] 诺氟沙星，氟哌酸

gastric/ˈgæstrɪk/ adj. 胃的，胃部的

endotoxin/ˌendoˈtɑksɪn/ n. 内毒素

exotoxin/ˌeksoʊˈtɒksɪn/ n. 外毒素

acidosis/ˌæsɪˈdoʊsɪs/ n. 酸液过多症，酸毒症，酸中毒

plasma/'plæzmə/ n. 血浆，原生质，细胞质，乳清

secretion/sɪ'kriːʃn/ n. 分泌，分泌物，藏匿，隐藏

electrolyte/ɪ'lektrəlaɪt/ n. ［化］电解液，电解质

spasm/'spæzəm/ n. 痉挛，抽搐，（能量、行为等的）突发，发作

renal/'riːnl/ adj. 肾脏的

gastric acid 胃酸

1.2.2 流行性出血热 Hemorrhagic fever with renal syndrome

流行性出血热又称肾综合征出血热，是由布尼亚病毒科汉坦病毒属的各型病毒引起的、以鼠类为主要传染源的一种自然疫源性疾病。该病主要分布在欧亚大陆，但汉坦病毒几乎遍布世界各大洲。

Hemorrhagic fever with renal syndrome (HFRS) is a group of clinically similar illnesses caused by hantaviruses from the family Bunyaviridae and is a kind of natural epidemic disease mainly infected by mice. It is mainly distributed in Eurasia, but hantaviruses are found throughout the world.

1. 临床表现

最初症状突然，包括头痛、发热、寒战、恶心、背痛、腹痛、视力模糊、脸部潮红、眼睛发红或皮疹。随后出现低血压、急性休克、血管渗漏出血、急性肾功能衰竭等症状。

1. Clinical features

Initial symptoms begin suddenly and include intense headaches, fever, chills, nausea, back and abdominal pain, and blurred vision. Patients may have flushing of the face, redness or inflammation of the eyes, or a rash. Later symptoms can include low blood pressure, acute shock, vascular leakage, and acute kidney failure.

2. 潜伏期

流行性出血热的症状通常在接触感染物后 1~2 周出现，极少数为 8 周。

3. 传播途径

汉坦病毒主要通过啮齿动物携带及传播。人接触携带病毒的尿液、排泄物、唾液、来自洞穴的尘埃等而染病。人被感染的老鼠咬伤或通过破损的皮肤伤口、眼睛黏膜、鼻子、嘴巴等直接接触病毒污染的尿液或者其他物质亦可致感染。人传人可能发生，但极少见。

4. 预防措施

旅行前，应向医生了解目的地该病流行情况。

旅行时，应避免接触啮齿动物的尿、排泄物、唾液和洞穴物料等，清除啮齿动物污染区域时要做好个人防护措施。

旅行回国入境时或入境后，如出现相关症状，应尽早就医并主动告知医生近期旅行情况。

2. Incubation period

Symptoms of HFRS usually develop within 1 to 2 weeks after exposure to infectious material. In rare cases, they may take up to 8 weeks to develop.

3. Route of transmission

Hantaviruses are carried and transmitted by rodents. People can be infected after exposure to aerosolized urine, droppings, saliva of infected rodents or dust from the nests. Transmission may also occur when infected urine or other materials are directly introduced into broken skin or onto the mucous membranes of the eyes, nose, or mouth. Transmission from person to person may occur, but is extremely rare.

4. Prevention measures

Consult a doctor the epidemic situation of the destination before travel.

While traveling, avoid contact with rodent urine, droppings, saliva, and nesting materials, and take safety measures when cleaning rodent-infested areas.

See a doctor and tell him/her your recent travel history if there is sudden onset of relative symptoms after travel.

Words & Expressions

abdominal/æb'dɑːmɪn（ə）l/ adj. 腹部的

inflammation/ˌɪnfləˈmeɪʃn/ n. ［医］炎症，燃烧，发火

rodent/'rodnt/ n. 啮齿目动物（如老鼠等）

urine/'jʊrɪn/ n. 尿，小便，下泉

saliva/səˈlaɪvə/ n. 唾液，口水，津，吐沫，涎

mucous/'mjuːkəs/ adj. 黏液的，黏液覆盖的

membrane/'membren/ n.（动植物的）膜，（可起防水、防风等作用的）膜状物

the mucous membranes　黏膜

1.2.3　手足口病　Hand，foot and mouth disease

手足口病是一种常见于儿童的疾病，通常由肠道病毒如柯萨奇病毒和肠病毒71型引起。肠病毒71型引致的手足口病备受关注，是因为它较有可能引致严重并发症（如病毒性脑膜炎、脑炎、类小儿麻痹瘫痪），甚至死亡。在我国南方，手足口病的高峰期一般为初夏至秋季，亦有机会于冬季出现小高峰。

1. 临床表现

大部分患者症状轻微并在

Hand, foot and mouth disease(HFMD) is a common disease in children caused by enteroviruses such as coxsackieviruses and enterovirus 71(EV71). The EV71 infection is of particular concern as it more likely associates with severe outcomes(like viral meningitis, encephalitis, poliomyelitis-like paralysis) and even death. The usual peak season for HFMD in south China is from early summer to autumn and a smaller peak may also occur in winter.

1. Clinical features

The disease is mostly self-limiting and

7～10 天内自行痊愈。病发初期，通常会出现发烧、食欲不振、疲倦和喉咙痛。发烧后一至两天，口腔黏膜出现散在的疱疹或溃疡。疱疹和溃疡通常位于舌头、牙肉以及口腔的两腮内侧。亦会出现不痒及有时会带有小水疱的红疹。手、足、臀部、腿部出现斑丘疹，后转为疱疹，疱疹周围可有炎性红晕，疱内液体较少。手足部较多，掌背面均有。消退后不留痕迹，无色素沉着。

患者痊愈后会对相应的肠病毒产生抗体。但日后仍可感染由其他肠病毒引致的手足口病。尚无药物治疗手足口病。

2. 潜伏期

约 3～7 天。

3. 传播途径

手足口病主要通过接触患者的鼻或喉咙分泌物、唾液、穿破的水疱或粪便，或触摸受污染的物件而传播。患者在病发首周最具传染性，而病毒可

resolves in 7 to 10 days. It usually begins with fever, poor appetite, tiredness, and sore throat. One or two days after fever onset, scattered herpes or ulcers develop in the mouth. They are usually located on the tongue, gum, and inside of the cheeks. There may also be non-itchy skin rash, some with blisters. Spot papule may occur in hand, foot, hip, leg and then turn for herpes. There can be inflammatory redness around herpes with less fluid. They are more in hands and feet, both in palm and back. There is no scar and pigmentation left after the herpes subside.

Infection will result in immunity to (protection against) the specific virus that has caused HFMD. However, a second attack of HFMD may occur following infection with a different member of the enterovirus group. There is no specific drug treatment for HFMD.

2. Incubation period

About 3 to 7 days.

3. Route of transmission

The disease mainly spreads by contact with an infected person's nose or throat discharges, saliva, fluid from vesicles or stool, or after touching contaminated objects. The disease is most contagious

在其粪便中存活数星期。

4. 预防措施

目前仍未有疫苗可有效预防手足口病。因此，良好的个人及环境卫生习惯最为重要。

患者应多喝水，保持充足休息，同时亦可用药物对症治疗，以舒缓发烧和口腔溃疡引致的痛楚。

为免把病毒传染给别人，患病的儿童应该避免上学或参加集体活动，直至所有水疱结痂。如感染是由肠病毒71型引致，患者完全康复（即发烧及红疹消退，以及所有水疱结痂）后应居家多休息两周再回校上课。

父母要细心观察儿童的病情。如出现持续高烧、神情呆滞或病情恶化等情况，应立即求医。

用清水及肥皂液洗手，尤其是在接触鼻和口前，进食或处理食物前，接触水疱后，如厕后，当手被呼吸道分泌物污染时，更换尿片后，或处理被污染的物件后。

during the first week of the illness and the viruses can be found in stool for weeks.

4. Prevention measures

There is no effective vaccine. Good personal and environmental hygiene is the mainstay of prevention.

Patients should drink plenty of water and take adequate rest and may receive symptomatic treatment to reduce fever and pain from oral ulcers.

Sick children should stay away from school or gatherings till all vesicles have dried up to avoid spreading the disease. If infection is caused by enterovirus 71 (EV71), the patient should stay at home for two more weeks after recovery from the disease (i. e. fever and rash have subsided, and vesicles have dried).

Parents should monitor the child's condition closely and seek medical advice immediately if persistent high fever, decrease in alertness or deterioration in general condition develops.

Wash hands with liquid soap and water especially before touching nose and mouth, before eating or handling food, after touching blister, after using toilet, or when hands are contaminated by respiratory secretions, after changing diapers, or after handling soiled articles.

打喷嚏或咳嗽时，用纸巾掩盖口鼻。将染污的纸巾弃置于有盖垃圾箱内。

Cover both nose and mouth with tissue paper when coughing or sneezing and discard the soiled tissue paper in a lidded rubbish bin.

不要共用毛巾及其他个人物品。

Do not share towels and other personal items.

经常清洁和消毒常接触的表面，如家具、玩具和共用物件。

Regularly clean and disinfect frequently touched surface such as furniture, toys and commonly shared items.

当学校或院舍暴发手足口病期间，避免集体活动。此外，应减少人手调动，尽量安排同一组员工照顾同一组学生。

Avoid group activities when HFMD outbreak occurs in the school or institution. Besides, minimise staff movement and arrange the same group of staff to take care of the same group of children as far as possible.

避免与患者有亲密接触，如接吻、拥抱。

Avoid close contact (such as kissing, hugging) with infected persons.

Words & Expressions

enterovirus/ˌentərəʊˈvaɪrəs/ n. 肠道病毒

meningitis/ˌmenɪnˈdʒaɪtɪs/ n. 脑膜炎

encephalitis/enˌsefəˈlaɪtɪs/ n. 脑炎

poliomyelitis/ˌpolɪoˌmaɪəˈlaɪtɪs/ n. 脊髓灰质炎，小儿麻痹症

paralysis/pəˈræləsɪs/ n. 麻痹，瘫痪，中风，无能，无气力

ulcer/ˈʌlsər/ n. [医] 溃疡，腐烂物，道德败坏，腐败

gum/gʌm/ n. 口香糖，树胶，黏胶，牙龈

blister/ˈblɪstər/ n. 水疱，水肿，疱，气泡

papule/ˈpæpjuːl/ n. 丘疹，长疮，小乳头

herpes/ˈhɜːrpiːz/ n. ［医］疱疹

pigmentation/ˌpɪgmenˈteɪʃn/ n. 染色，着色，色素沉着

vesicle/ˈvesɪkl/ n. 囊，泡，小泡，［医］痘，水疱

diaper/ˈdaɪpər/ n. 有菱形花格的麻或棉织物，尿布

mainstay/ˈmeɪnsteɪ/ n. 支柱，柱石，骨干，中流砥柱，主要的依靠

poliomyelitis-like paralysis　脊髓灰质炎样瘫痪/麻痹

1.2.4 轮状病毒感染　Rotavirus infection

轮状病毒感染主要见于婴幼儿，全世界每年因轮状病毒感染导致的婴幼儿死亡的人数大约为 90 万人，其中大多数发生在发展中国家。在我国，每年大约有 1000 万婴幼儿患轮状病毒感染性胃肠炎，占婴幼儿人数的四分之一，是引起婴幼儿严重腹泻的最主要原因。婴幼儿感染者病情一般较重，病死率高。近年口服补液的使用显著降低了因腹泻所致的死亡。

1. 病原体

轮状病毒总共有 7 种，分别以英文字母 A-G 编号。人类主要感染轮状病毒 A 种和 B 种，感染后主要侵犯人体空肠

Rotavirus infection is mainly found in infants and can cause dealths of 900,000 infants worldwide each year; most of them are in developing countries. In China, about 10 million infants suffer from rotavirus gastroenteritis, which is the most important cause of severe diarrhea, accounting for 1/4 of the infant population every year. Infantile infections are generally severe and have a high fatality rate. The use of oral rehydration has significantly reduced deaths from diarrhea in recent years.

1. Pathogens

There are seven types of rotaviruses, each numbered A-G. Humans are mainly infected with rotavirus A and B, which mainly invade human jejunum microvillus

微绒毛上皮细胞，使其凋亡，导致小肠功能丧失，引起腹泻等。

2. 临床表现

急性发热；呕吐及腹泻，大便黄色水样；全身酸痛、乏力。

3. 传染源

病人和隐性感染者是本病的主要传染源。

4. 传播途径

病人及隐性感染者的粪便污染水源或食物后引起传播。

5. 易感人群

多见于5岁以下儿童。

6. 预防措施

在日常生活中，应注重个人卫生，尤其要加强对婴幼儿的手卫生护理。

母亲在哺乳前应注意乳头的清洁卫生，用奶瓶喂奶时，应注意奶瓶奶头的消毒。

儿童发生腹泻时，家长应积极配合医生治疗，饮食应以清淡为主，保证儿童的营养供给和身体所需。

epithelial cells and cause apoptosis, resulting in loss of small intestine function and diarrhea.

2. Clinical features

Acute fever; vomiting and diarrhea, with yellow and watery stool; body aches, fatigue.

3. Source of infection

Patients and inapparent infected people are the main source of infection.

4. Route of transmission

Through water or food polluted by feces of patients and latent infected persons.

5. Susceptible population

Most common in children under 5 years old.

6. Prevention measures

Pay attention to personal hygiene, especially to strengthening hand hygiene care of infants in daily life.

Mothers should take care to clean the nipple before breastfeeding and disinfect bottle nipple when feeding with bottle.

Once children have diarrhea, parents should actively cooperate with doctors for treatment. The diet should be light to ensure the nutritional supply and physical needs for children.

在流行季节要尽量少去公共场合或空气不流通的地方，家里也要注意保持干净卫生和空气流通，减少病毒、细菌的滋生。

对一些身体虚弱的儿童，特别是早产儿或患有先天性心脏病等先天性疾病的儿童，也可在流行季节先行口服轮状病毒疫苗，以减少发病的可能性。

Avoid going to crowded or poorly ventilated places in epidemic season. Keep the home clean and maintain good ventilation to reduce the breeding of viruses and bacteria.

Some frail children, especially those who are premature or have congenital diseases such as congenital heart disease, can also take the rotavirus vaccine orally in advance to reduce the likelihood of illness in epidemic season.

Words & Expressions

rotavirus/ˌroʊtə'vaɪrəs/ n. 轮状病毒

rehydration/ˌrihaɪ'dreʃən/ n. 再水化，再水合，补液

jejunum/dʒɪ'dʒuːnəm/ n. 空肠

villus/'vɪləs/ n. 绒毛，长茸毛

gastroenteritis/ˌgæstroʊˌentə'raɪtɪs/ n. 肠胃炎，胃肠炎

frail/freɪl/ adj. 脆弱的，虚弱的，意志薄弱的，易损的，易碎的

congenital/kən'dʒenɪtl/ adj. 先天的，天生的，先天性

microvillus/ˌmaɪkroʊ'vɪləs/ n. 微绒毛

1.2.5　诺如病毒感染　Norovirus infection

诺如病毒感染在全世界范围内均有流行，全年均可发生

Norovirus infection is endemic worldwide and can occur throughout the

感染，感染对象主要是成人和学龄儿童，寒冷季节呈现高发。常在幼儿园、学校和养老院等人员密集的场所引起聚集性疫情。

1. 病原体

诺如病毒，又称诺瓦克病毒，是人类杯状病毒科（HuCV）中诺如病毒属的一种病毒，是一组形态相似、抗原性略有不同的病毒颗粒。

2. 临床表现

人感染诺如病毒后可导致急性胃肠炎，主要症状有呕吐、腹泻、恶心、腹痛。部分患者有头痛、发热、寒战、肌肉疼痛等症状，通常持续 2~3 天。诺如病毒急性胃肠炎为自限性疾病，病情轻微，无后遗症，但老人、婴幼儿及患有基础性疾病的人发生严重并发症的风险较高，需特别关注。目前诺如病毒急性胃肠炎没有特效药物，以对症治疗为主。

year, mainly among adults and school-age children, with a high incidence in cold seasons. It often causes clusters of outbreaks in kindergartens, schools, nursing homes and other crowded places.

1. Pathogens

Norovirus, also known as Norwalk viruses, is a virus of genus *Noroviruses* in Human Calicivirus family （HuCV）. Norovirus is a group of virus particles with similar morphology and slightly different antigenicity.

2. Clinical features

Norovirus can cause acute gastroenteritis in humans. The main symptoms include vomiting, diarrhea, nausea, and abdominal pain. Some patients have headache, fever, chills, muscle pain and other symptoms, which usually last for 2 to 3 days. Norovirus acute gastroenteritis is a self-limiting disease with mild symptoms and has no sequelae, but the elderly, infants and people with underlying diseases are at higher risk of serious complications, requiring special attention. At present, there is no specific drug for norovirus acute gastroenteritis, and therapeutic options are mainly symptomatic treatment.

3. 潜伏期

潜伏期为 24~48 小时。

4. 传染源

病人和病毒携带者。

5. 传播途径

可通过污染的食物、水传播，也可经接触病人排泄物或呕吐物，经污染的手、物体和用具，以及呕吐物产生的气溶胶等方式传播。牡蛎等双壳贝类可以富集海水中的诺如病毒，为高风险食物。另外，接触过诺如病毒感染患者，如照顾患者、与患者分享食物或共用餐具，也可增加感染风险。

6. 预防措施

注意个人卫生，饭前便后、加工食物之前要洗手。

生吃瓜果要洗净。牡蛎等贝类海产品必须充分加热煮熟后再吃。

要选用卫生合格的桶装水，喝开水。

如果家中出现诺如病毒急性胃肠炎患者，应使用患者自己的饮食用具及生活用品，尽

3. Incubation period

The incubation period is 24 to 48 hours.

4. Source of infection

Patients and carriers of the virus.

5. Route of transmission

It can spread through contaminated food and water, contact with the feces or vomit of sick people, contaminated hands, objects, utensils and aerosols produced by vomiting. Bivalve shellfish such as oyster can concentrate norovirus in seawater, which is a high-risk food. In addition, contact with a norovirus infected person, such as caring for a sick person, sharing food or cutlery, can also add the risk of being infected.

6. Prevention measures

Pay attention to personal hygiene. Wash hands before eating or processing food, or after using the toilet.

Clean the raw fruits before eating. Oysters and other shellfish must be fully heated and cooked before eating.

Choose qualified bottled water, and drink boiled water.

If a patient with norovirus acute gastroenteritis is at home, he/she should use his/her own eating utensils and daily

量不要与家人密切接触，患者发生呕吐或腹泻后，应及时消毒并清理排泄物。

托幼机构、学校等集体单位应加强传染病健康宣传工作，加强学校食品安全管理，提供安全饮用水，严格按照相关规定进行校内环境消毒工作。一旦发现儿童、学生出现聚集性恶心、呕吐、腹泻等症状，应及时向当地卫生部门报告，在相关专业人员指导下进行疫情调查和处置。

necessities, avoid close contact with his/her families as far as possible, and disinfect and clean up excrement in time after vomiting or diarrhea.

Kindergartens, schools, and other collective units should strengthen the health publicity of infectious diseases and management of school food safety, provid safe drinking water and strictly disinfect the school environment according to relevant regulations. Once children and students are found to have clustered nausea, vomiting, diarrhea and other symptoms, report to local health authorities in time and carry out epidemic investigation and treatment under the guidance of relevant professionals.

Words & Expressions

norovirus/'nɔːroʊvaɪrəs/ n. ［医］诺如病毒

calicivirus/kælɪsɪ'vaɪrəs/ n. 萼状病毒；（C-）［医］杯状病毒

morphology/mɔːr'fɑːlədʒi/ n. 形态学（尤指动植物形态学或词语形态学）

antigenicity/ˌæntidʒə'nisəti/ n. 抗原性

sequelae/sɪ'kwili/ n. 后继者，后遗症（sequela 的名词复数），并发症

utensil/ju'tensl/ n. （尤指厨房或家用的）器具，用具

feces/'fiːsiːz/ n. 粪，屎，渣滓，粪便

bivalve/'baɪvælv/ n. 双壳类，双阀

excrement/'ekskrɪmənt/ n. 排泄物（粪便），屎

oyster/'ɔɪstər/ n. 牡蛎，蚝

1.3 蚊媒传染病 Mosquito-borne infectious diseases

1.3.1 黄热病 Yellow fever

黄热病是由黄热病病毒引起的急性传染病，最初发现于非洲和美洲的热带地区。它主要通过伊蚊的叮咬来传播，感染人类和猴子。埃及伊蚊是主要传播媒介。黄热病会引起灾难性的疫情暴发，可通过大规模的疫苗接种来预防和控制。20世纪以来，该病在北美洲及欧洲未再发生，但在南美洲、非洲的一些国家和地区仍不时流行。

1. 病原体

黄热病病毒属于黄热病科黄热病毒属的病毒，为 RNA 病毒，具有嗜内脏性及嗜神经性，在室温下容易死亡。

2. 流行病学

黄热病是一种蚊媒性自然

Yellow fever is an acute infectious disease caused by yellow fever virus, found in tropical regions of Africa and the Americas. It principally affects humans and monkeys and is transmitted via the bite of Aedes mosquitoes. Aedes aegypti is the main vector. It can produce devastating outbreaks, which can be prevented and controlled by mass vaccination campaigns. The disease has not reappeared in North America and Europe since the 20th century, but it is still occasionally prevalent in South America, Africa and some countries and regions.

1. Pathogens

Yellow fever virus is a RNA virus belonging to the genus of yellow fever virus in yellow fever family. It is viscerotropic and neurotropic, and it easily dies at room temperature.

2. Epidemiology

Yellow fever is a mosquito-borne

疫源性疾病，流行模式可分为城市型和丛林型。丛林型是原发性自然疫源地，而城市型则是由于人类活动从前者扩散而致。

3. 传染源

城市型黄热病的主要传染源是患者和隐性感染者。丛林型黄热病的主要传染源是热带丛林中的猴子以及其他灵长类动物。

4. 传播途径

黄热病的主要传播媒介为埃及伊蚊。受感染的蚊可终身携带病毒，可经卵传递。

5. 易感人群

无免疫力的人群对黄热病普遍易感，隐性感染或发病后均能获得持久免疫力，其体内产生的中和抗体可保持终身，未发现再感染者。

6. 流行特征

城市型以"人—埃及伊

natural epidemic source disease. According to the epidemical patterns, it can be divided into urban yellow fever and jungle yellow fever. Jungle yellow fever is a primary natural foci disease, while urban yellow fever is caused by the spread of human activities from the former.

3. Source of infection

The main source of infection of urban yellow fever can be patients and latent infected persons. Jungle yellow fever is mainly transmitted by monkeys and the other primates living in the jungle.

4. Route of transmission

The main vector of yellow fever is Aedes mosquitoes. Infected mosquitoes can carry the viruses for lifetime and viruses can be transmitted through their ova.

5. Susceptible people

People with no immunity are generally susceptible to yellow fever, and can acquire lasting immunity either from latent infection or from the onset. The neutralization antibodies produced in their bodies can be maintained for lifetime, and no reinfected people have been found.

6. Epidemic characteristics

Urban yellow fever is transmitted by a cycle of person to Aedes aegypti, without a

蚊—人"形成循环，无贮存宿主；丛林型以"蚊—猴—蚊"形成循环，构成黄热病的自然疫源地。

7. 季节性

非洲和南美洲流行季节多在 3～4 月，此时雨多，湿度大，气温高，利于蚊媒滋生及病毒在蚊体内的繁殖。全年均可发病。

8. 临床表现

该病的最初症状通常在感染后 3～6 天出现。第一阶段，或称"急性"期的特征是发热、肌肉疼痛、头痛、寒战、食欲不振、恶心和呕吐。3～4 天后，大部分患者好转，症状消失。然而少数病例进入"毒性"期：再次发热，患者出现黄疸，有时出血，呕吐物中带血。大约 50% 进入毒性期的患者在 10～14 天内死亡。

9. 预防措施

目前该病尚无特效治疗方

reservoir host; while jungle yellow fever is transmitted by a cycle of mosquito to monkey, forming the natural foci of yellow fever.

7. Seasonality

The epidemic season in Africa and South America is from March to April. It is rainy with high humidity and temperature at this time, conducive to mosquito breeding and virus propagation in the mosquitoes. Yellow fever can occur throughout the whole year.

8. Clinical features

The first symptoms of the disease usually appear 3 to 6 days after infection. In the first, or "acute", phase is characterized by fever, muscle pain, headache, shivers, loss of appetite, nausea, and vomiting. After 3 to 4 days, most patients improve, and symptoms disappear. However, in a few cases, the disease enters a "toxic" phase: fever reappears, and the patient develops jaundice and sometimes bleeding, with blood appearing in the vomit. About 50% of patients who enter the toxic phase die within 10 to 14 days.

9. Prevention measures

There is no specific treatment for

法。强烈建议接种疫苗作为游客和该病流行国家当地居民的预防措施。

出国旅行前，可到当地海关了解前往国家/地区该病的流行情况，进行黄热病疫苗的预防接种。黄热病疫苗预防接种的免疫期自接种后第10日起终身有效。①

旅行时，应时常着长袖衣服和裤子，减少皮肤暴露；在外露的皮肤处涂驱蚊剂；住室内可用1%甲醚菊酯气雾剂或苯醚菊酯乳剂喷洒灭蚊。

旅行后，入境时向当地海关出示有效的黄热病预防接种证书。凡有突然发热、头痛等不适症状的病人，应主动申报并告知近期的旅行情况。

yellow fever. Vaccination is highly recommended as a preventive measure for travelers to and people living in endemic countries.

Before traveling abroad, you can consult the local customs about the epidemic situation of destination and get vaccination of yellow fever vaccine. The immune period of yellow fever vaccination is valid for lifetime from the 10th day after vaccination.

While traveling, wear long-sleeved clothes and trousers frequently to reduce skin exposure; use mosquito repellent on exposed skin; apply mosquito spraying indoors with 1% ether inulin aerosol or benzene ether inulin emulsion.

After travel, show the effective yellow fever vaccination certificate to the local customs officials. Patients with sudden fever, headache and other uncomfortable symptoms should take the initiative to declare and inform them of the recent travel situation.

---

① 根据《国际卫生条例》规定和世界卫生组织有关要求，黄热病疫苗接种属于强制性预防接种。来自黄热病流行区的人员，在入境时，必须向海关出示有效的黄热病预防接种证书。

Words & Expressions

mosquito/məˈskiːtoʊ/ n. 蚊子

mosquito-borne/məsˈkitoʊbˈɔn/ adj. 蚊传播的，蚊传染的，蚊媒的

aedes/eˈidiz/ n. 伊蚊（一种传染黄热病的蚊子）

viscerotropic/ˌvɪsərəˈtrɒpɪk/ adj.（病毒等）亲内脏的

ova/ˈoʊvə/ n. ［生］卵子，卵细胞（ovum 的名词复数）

vector/ˈvektər/ n. 矢量，航向，带菌者，载体

foci/ˈfəʊsaɪ/ n. 焦距，配光，焦点（focus 的名词复数），［医学］病灶，疫源地

propagation/ˌprɑːpəˈgeɪʃn/ n. 传播，蔓延，波及深度

jaundice/ˈdʒɔːndɪs/ n. 黄疸病，偏见

repellent/rɪˈpelənt/ n. 反拨力，排拒力，防水布，防水剂，驱虫剂，消肿药

ether/ˈiːθər/ n. ［化］醚；苍穹，苍天，太空

inulin/ɪnjəlɪn/ n. 菊

ether inulin 乙醚菊粉

1.3.2 登革热 Dengue fever

登革热在热带和亚热带地区广泛传播，目前在非洲、美洲、东地中海、东南亚和西太平洋的 100 多个国家呈地方性流行，东南亚和西太平洋地区受影响最为严重。仅在 2007 年，美洲就有 89 万多登革热报告病例，其中 26 万为登革出血

Dengue fever is widespread in tropical and subtropical regions and is currently endemic in more than 100 countries in Africa, the Americas, the Eastern Mediterranean, Southeast Asia, and the Western Pacific. The hardest-hit countries and regions are in Southeast Asia and the Western Pacific. Only in 2007, more than

热病例。世界卫生组织估计，每年世界上有5000万登革热感染病例，50万人因患登革出血热需住院治疗。登革出血热有较高的病死率，出现休克者，病死率可高达10%~40%。

1. 临床表现

登革热是一种急性发热性传染病，引起该病的病原体为登革病毒，登革病毒通过蚊子传播。登革热发病较急，主要表现为突然起病、高热、头痛、全身肌肉和关节疼痛、乏力、颜面潮红、结膜充血，并可以出现消化道症状，皮肤出现皮疹、出血点。

2. 传染源

患者和隐性感染者为主要传染源。

3. 传播途径

登革热通过蚊媒传播，最主要的是埃及伊蚊和白纹伊蚊。

890,000 cases of dengue fever were reported in the Americas, of which 260,000 were cases of dengue hemorrhagic fever. WHO estimates there may be 50 million dengue infections worldwide each year, with 500,000 cases requiring hospitalization for dengue hemorrhagic fever. Dengue hemorrhagic fever has a high fatality rate, which can be as high as 10% to 40% in cases of shock.

1. Clinical features

Dengue fever is an acute febrile infectious disease, characterized by sudden onset, high fever, headache, anorexia, myalgia, gastrointestinal disturbances, petechia and rash. Dengue fever is caused by dengue virus, which is transmitted by the bite of mosquitoes.

2. Source of infection

Patients and latent infections can be the main source of infection.

3. Route of transmission

Dengue fever is transmitted by mosquitoes, most notably Aedes aegypti and Aedes albopictus.

4. 易感人群

在新流行区人群普遍易感。

5. 预防措施

穿长袖衫及长裤；用驱蚊剂涂在身体外露部分；当室内无空调时要用隔蚊帘或蚊帐；避免逗留在丛林地区。

出国人员可到当地海关了解国外疫情并采取相应预防措施。

如果旅客来自登革热流行国家或地区，并且在15天内出现发热或其他不适，入境时请主动向当地海关报告。

4. Susceptible population

People in new epidemic areas are generally susceptible.

5. Prevention measures

Wear long-sleeved shirts and trousers; use insect repellents containing DEET on exposed skin; use bed-nets if sleeping areas are not air-conditioned; avoid staying in the jungle for a long time.

Consult for epidemic situation of destination from local customs and take the corresponding preventive measures.

If you came from the epidemic regions of dengue fever and had fever or other discomforts within 15 days, please contact the local customs when you entered China.

Words & Expressions

febrile/ˈfiːbraɪl/ adj. 发热的

anorexia/ˌænəˈreksiə/ n. 厌食症，厌食，食欲缺乏，胃呆

petechia/pɪˈtikɪr/ n. 瘀点

DEET/diːt/ n. 避蚊胺（一种驱蚊剂）

aedes albopictus 白纹伊蚊

1.3.3 基孔肯雅热 Chikungunya fever

基孔肯雅热是一种始发于非洲的病毒性传染病，1952年首次在坦桑尼亚流行。基孔肯雅热主要分布于冬季气温18℃以上的非洲和东南亚热带及亚热带地区。据世界卫生组织报道，近年来非洲和东南亚地区常发生基孔肯雅热的流行和暴发。1965年，印度发生大流行，30万人感染，在缅甸、泰国、柬埔寨、越南、印度尼西亚和马来西亚等东南亚国家都有流行。2006年以来，在斯里兰卡、马尔代夫、加蓬、意大利、印度、印度尼西亚、新加坡等国家有基孔肯雅热疾病流行的报道。在中国、美国、德国等国家也有输入性基孔肯雅热患者的报告。基孔肯雅热的病死率不高。

1. 病原体

基孔肯雅热是由基孔肯雅病毒引起的急性传染病，病毒

Chikungunya fever is a viral infection that originated in Africa and first emerged in Tanzania in 1952. Chikungunya fever is mainly distributed in tropical and subtropical regions of Africa and Southeast Asia with winter temperature above 18℃. According to the World Health Organization, epidemics and outbreaks of chikungunya fever have frequently occurred in Africa and Southeast Asia in recent years. In 1965, a pandemic occurred in India, with 300,000 people infected. It was also prevalent in Myanmar, Thailand, Cambodia, Vietnam, Indonesia, Malaysia, and other Southeast Asian countries. Chikungunya fever has been reported in Sri Lanka, Maldives, Gabon, Italy, India, Indonesia, Singapore, and other countries since 2006. Imported chikungunya fever cases have also been reported in China, USA, and Germany. The mortality rate of chikungunya fever is not high.

1. Pathogens

Chikungunya fever is an acute infectious disease caused by chikungunya

进入细胞后，在细胞内复制，导致细胞坏死和凋亡，严重者可出现脑膜脑炎、肝功能损伤、心肌炎及皮肤黏膜出血。

2. 临床表现

基孔肯雅热的主要症状有突然发热、寒战、躯干部皮疹、严重关节痛和头痛等，可伴有恶心、呕吐、畏光、结膜充血、腹痛或出血症状。

3. 传播途径

基孔肯雅热的传播媒介主要是埃及伊蚊、白纹伊蚊等伊蚊属。其中埃及伊蚊为家栖蚊种，是传播基孔肯雅病毒能力最强的蚊种；白纹伊蚊是引起近期印度洋岛屿基孔肯雅热流行的主要媒介，该蚊种在我国分布较为广泛。

4. 预防措施

防蚊灭蚊工作是预防和控制该传染病的关键措施。具体的预防性措施包括清除积水等蚊虫滋生地，使用蚊帐，穿着

virus. After entering cells, the virus replicates in these cells, leading to cell necrosis and apoptosis. Patients can develop meningoencephalitis, liver function injury, myocarditis, and skin mucous membrane hemorrhage.

2. Clinical features

The main symptoms of chikungunya fever are sudden fever, chills, trunk rash, severe joint pain, and headache, accompanied by nausea, vomiting, photophobia, conjunctival congestion, abdominal pain, or bleeding.

3. Route of transmission

Mosquitoes are the main vectors of chikungunya fever, which include Aedes aegypti and Aedes albopictus. Among them, Aedes aegypti is a kind of domestic mosquito species, which has the strongest ability to transmit chikungunya virus. Aedes albopictus is the main vector causing the recent epidemic of chikungunya fever in the Indian Ocean islands, which is widely distributed in China.

4. Prevention measures

Mosquito control is a key measure to prevent the infectious disease. The specific preventive measures include removing water in mosquito infested areas, using mosquito

长袖衣物或涂抹驱蚊剂防止蚊虫叮咬等。

nets, wearing long sleeve clothes, or applying mosquito repellent to prevent mosquito bites.

5. 入出境提示

旅客如果赴非洲、东南亚地区旅游，要注意预防蚊虫叮咬，一旦出现上述症状应及时就医。途经上述地区入境的旅客，若出现发热等症状，请在入境时主动向海关检疫岗申报。赴上述目的地的旅客请做好自我防护，并做好各项应急准备工作。

5. Entry and exit reminds

Passengers who travel to Africa and Southeast Asia should pay attention to preventing from mosquito biting, and see a doctor in time if the above symptoms appeared. Passengers who enter China through the above-mentioned areas should take the initiative to declare to the customs quarantine post if fever and other symptoms appeared. Passengers to the above destinations should do a good job in self-protection and emergency preparations.

Words & Expressions

chikungunya/ˌtʃɪkʊŋˈɡʊnjə/ n. 基孔肯雅热

Tanzania/ˌtænzəˈniə/ n. 坦桑尼亚

Cambodia/kæmˈboʊdiə/ n. 柬埔寨

1.3.4 疟疾 Malaria

疟疾是国际监测的传染病之一，也是世界六大热带病之一，广泛流行于世界各地，主要在亚洲、非洲及拉丁美洲的国家和地区流行。每年全球疟疾发病人数 1.5 亿到 3 亿，数十万人因疟疾死亡。根据世界卫生组织数据，2020 年估计有 2.41 亿疟疾病例，死亡人数估计为 62.7 万。氯喹为控制发作和预防疟疾的首选药物。间日疟、三日疟经治疗预后较好，大多痊愈。恶性疟发作凶险，如脑型疟，国外报道接受治疗病人的病死率为 22%。

Malaria is one of the infectious diseases of international surveillance and one of the six major tropical diseases in the world, which is widely epidemic all over the world, mainly in Asia, Africa, and Latin America. 150 million to 300 million people are infected with malaria, and hundreds of thousands of people die each year. According to the WHO, in 2020, there were an estimated 241 million cases of malaria worldwide. The estimated number of malaria deaths stood at 627, 000 in 2020. Chloroquine is the first choice medicine for malaria control and prevention. Patients infected with plasmodium vivax and plasmodium malaria have a good prognosis after treatment and are mostly cured. Falciparum malaria is a dangerous disease, such as cerebral malaria, and the fatality rate of the patients under treatment is 22%, according to foreign reports.

1. 病原体

疟疾是由疟原虫引起的寄生虫病，寄生于人体的疟原虫有四种：间日疟原虫、恶性疟

1. Pathogens

Malaria is a parasitic disease caused by plasmodium, four kinds of which parasitic in the human body are plasmodium vivax,

原虫、三日疟原虫和卵形疟原虫。在我国以前两种为常见，疟疾主要导致患者溶血性贫血、凝血功能障碍，严重者可导致肝功能障碍、急性肾功能障碍等。目前对子孢子疫苗的免疫、子孢子疫苗和子代配子体疫苗的研究有重要进展，但到目前为止还没有安全有效的疟疾疫苗用于实际应用。

2. 临床表现

疟疾的三个基本症状为周期性发热、贫血和脾肿大。潜伏期是指在疟疾发作之前孢子虫侵入人体的时间。疟疾是一种周期性发热、癫痫发作（发冷、发热、出汗、发热）。潜伏期取决于被感染的疟原虫的类型。

疟疾通常有以下四种临床症状：

前驱期：头痛、身体疼痛、疲劳、发冷。

发冷期：脚冷，然后颤抖、发冷，嘴唇和指甲苍白，发绀。

plasmodium falciparum, plasmodium malaria and plasmodium ovale. The first two plasmodia are common in China. Malaria mainly causes hemolytic anemia and coagulation dysfunction, and can even lead to liver dysfunction and acute renal dysfunction in severe cases. At present, there has been significant progress in the research of sporozoite vaccine immunization, sporosporal vaccine and progametophyte vaccine. But so far no malaria vaccine is safe and effective for practical application.

2. Clinical features

There are three basic symptoms of malaria: periodic fever, anemia, and splenomegaly. Incubation period refers to the time when sporozoites invade the body before malaria onset. Malaria is a kind of periodic fever and seizures (chills, fever, sweating, fever). The incubation period varies depending on the kind of plasmodium persons infected.

Malaria usually has four clinical symptoms as follows：

Prodromal stage: headache, body aches, fatigue, chills.

Cold stage: cold feet, then shaking, chills, pale lips and nails, cyanosis. The

体温迅速上升，持续 10 分钟至 2 小时以上。

发热期：寒战、发热、头痛、口渴，体温可上升至 39℃ 以上，有的患者可抽搐，此期持续 2~3 小时。

出汗期：发高烧出汗后，体温迅速下降，此期持续 1 小时以上。

3. 潜伏期

疟疾的潜伏期为 3~30 天。恶性疟平均 12 天，间日疟和卵形疟平均 14 天，但间日疟有时可能超过 12 个月。经输血传播疟疾，潜伏期一般为 7~14 天。

4. 传染源

疟疾病人及疟原虫携带者是疟疾的传染源。

5. 传播途径

疟疾的自然传播媒介是按蚊，另外输入带疟原虫的血液也可传播疟疾。

6. 易感人群

人群普遍易感。

body temperature rises rapidly and lasts for 10 minutes to 2 hours.

Fever stage: chills, fever, headache and thirst. The body temperature can rise to 39℃ or more, and some patients can twitch. It lasts for 2 to 3 hours.

Sweating stage: sweating after high fever, body temperature droping rapidly. It may lasts for more than 1 hours.

3. Incubation period

The incubation period of malaria is from 3 to 30 days. The incubation period of falciparum malaria averages 12 days, and that of vivax malaria and oval malaria averages 14 days, but that of vivax malaria sometimes can be more than 12 months. If malaria is transmitted by blood transfusion, the incubation period is usually 7 to 14 days.

4. Source of infection

Malaria patients and plasmodium carriers can be the source of malaria infection.

5. Route of transmission

The natural vector of malaria is Anopheles mosquitoes, and transfusions of plasmodium blood can transmit malaria.

6. Susceptible population

People are generally susceptible.

7. 预防措施

要加强健康教育，使群众了解疟疾知识，自觉配合防治工作。加强对疟疾流行地区旅行者和无免疫力人群的健康指导。

加强个人预防。提倡使用蚊帐、蚊香、青蒿植物、烟熏、驱虫剂。必要时使用驱虫剂以防止蚊虫叮咬。

7. Prevention measures

Health education should be strengthened so as to enable the masses to understand malaria knowledge and consciously cooperate in the prevention work. Strengthen health guidance for travelers in the malaria endemic areas and people without immunity.

Strengthen individual prevention. The use of mosquito nets, mosquito coils, artemisia, smoke, insect repellent is recommended. Try to use insect repellents to prevent mosquito bites if necessary.

Words & Expressions

malaria/mə'leriə/ n. 疟疾

malarial/mə'leriəl/ adj. 患疟疾的，毒气的

plasmodium/plæz'modɪəm/ n. 原形体，变形体，疟原虫

vivax/'vaivæks/ n. 疟原虫（指引起疟疾的单细胞动物）

anopheles/ə'nɑːfəliz/ n. （传布疟疾寄生虫的）按蚊

parasite/'pærəˌsaɪt/ n. 寄生植物（或动物），寄生虫，不劳而获者

hemolytic/hiː'mɑːlɪtɪk/ adj. ［医］溶血的

anemia/ə'nimiə/ n. 贫血症，无活力，无生气

splenomegaly/ˌspleno'megəli/ n. 脾（肿）大，脾肿大，巨脾

sporozoite/ˌspoʊrə'zoʊaɪt/ n. 孢子体，子孢子

artemisia/ˌɑrtɪ'mɪzɪə/ n. 蒿属植物

falciparum malaria 恶性疟疾

plasmodium vivax 疟原虫

1.3.5 日本脑炎 Japanese encephalitis

日本脑炎又名"流行性乙型脑炎",是一种经由蚊子传播的疾病。此病由日本脑炎病毒引致,经带病毒的蚊子叮咬而感染。日本脑炎的主要病媒蚊是三带喙库蚊。日本脑炎主要流行于亚洲及西太平洋地区的郊外及农村。

Japanese encephalitis (also known as epidemic encephalitis B) is a mosquito-borne disease caused by the Japanese encephalitis virus. The virus is transmitted by the bites of infected mosquitoes. The principal type of mosquito that transmits the disease is called Culex tritaeniorhynchus. The disease occurs mainly in the rural and agricultural areas of Asia and the Western Pacific region.

1. 临床表现

日本脑炎从受到感染至发病一般为 4~14 天,病情轻微者除发烧及头痛外,一般不会有其他显著病征。病情严重者则进展较快,并出现头痛、发高烧、颈部僵硬、神志不清、昏迷、震颤、抽搐(尤其是幼童)及瘫痪等症状。

1. Clinical features

Symptoms usually start at around 4 to 14 days after being infected. Mild infections may not have apparent symptoms other than fever or headache. More severe infection is marked by quick onset of headache, high fever, neck stiffness, impaired mental state, coma, tremors, convulsions (especially in children) and paralysis.

2. 传播途径

蚊子于稻田等有大量积水的地方繁殖,叮咬带病毒的猪或野生雀鸟后受到感染,再叮咬人类或动物时将病毒传播。此病不会直接人传人。

2. Route of transmission

The infected mosquitoes transmit the virus to humans and animals through biting. The mosquitoes breed where there is abundant water such as rice paddies and become infected by feeding on pigs and wild birds infected with the Japanese encephalitis virus. The disease is not directly transmitted from person to person.

3. 治疗方法与并发症

日本脑炎并无特定的治疗方法。医生一般对患者施以支持性治疗。出现病症的患者病死率可高达30%。康复者中也会有20%~30%出现如瘫痪、反复抽搐或失语等永久性智力、行为或神经问题。

4. 疫苗

由于日本脑炎疫苗的接种，在中国的部分地区、日本、韩国，以及尼泊尔、斯里兰卡、泰国和越南，日本脑炎的个案已经在下降中。疫苗适用于准备前往日本脑炎流行区（尤其是当地郊区）并逗留一个月或以上的游客；对于一些短期旅游（不足一个月），旅客如果计划于疾病传播季节到郊区并大部分时间进行户外或夜间活动，亦应接种疫苗。

5. 预防措施

预防日本脑炎，应采取防蚊措施，避免被蚊子叮咬。传播日本脑炎病毒的蚊子于黄昏

3. Treatment and complications

There is no specific treatment for this disease. Supportive therapy is indicated. The case-fatality rate can be as high as 30% among those with symptoms. Of those who survive, 20% to 30% suffer permanent intellectual, behavioral or neurological problems such as paralysis, recurrent seizures or inability to speak.

4. Vaccines

The incidence of Japanese encephalitis has been declining in some regions of China, in Japan, the Republic of Korea, Nepal, Sri Lanka, Thailand, and Vietnam, largely as a result of vaccination. Vaccination is recommended for travelers who plan to stay one month or longer in endemic areas, particularly in rural areas, and for short-term(less than one month) travelers if they plan to have significant extensive outdoor or night-time exposure in rural areas during the transmission season of the disease.

5. Prevention measures

To prevent the disease, one should take general measures to prevent mosquito bites and avoid going to rural areas from

至黎明时分最为活跃，因此这段时间应避免前往郊外。准备前往此病流行地区的人士，更应加倍注意。

穿着宽松、浅色的长袖上衣及长裤，并于外露的皮肤及衣服涂上含避蚊胺（DEET）成分的昆虫驱避剂。

户外活动时采取其他的防护措施。避免使用有香味的化妆品或护肤品。依照指示重复使用昆虫驱避剂。

如果打算前往相关疾病流行的地区或国家，应在出发前6周或更早咨询医生，并采取额外的预防措施，避免受到叮咬。

如到流行地区的郊外旅行，应带便携式蚊帐，并在蚊帐上使用氯菊酯（一种杀虫剂）。切勿将氯菊酯涂在皮肤上。如感到不适，应尽快就医。

旅游人士若感到身体不适，如发烧，应尽快就医，并将行程细节告知医生。

dusk till dawn when the mosquitoes spreading this virus are most active. People planning to travel to areas in which Japanese encephalitis is endemic should take special note.

Wear loose, light-colored, long-sleeved tops and trousers, and put DEET-containing insect repellent on exposed parts of the body and clothing.

Take additional preventive measures when engaging in outdoor activities. Avoid using fragrant cosmetics or skin care products. Re-apply insect repellents according to instructions.

If going to affected areas or countries, travelers should arrange a consultation with doctor at least 6 weeks before the trip and take extra preventive measures to avoid mosquito bite.

During the trip, if travelling in endemic rural areas, travelers should carry a portable bed net and apply permethrin(an insecticide) on it. Permethrin should not be applied to skin. Seek medical advice promptly if feeling unwell.

Travelers if feeling unwell, e. g. running a fever, should seek medical advice promptly, and provide travel details to the doctor.

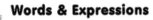

Words & Expressions

tremor/'tremər/ n.（身体或声音的）颤抖，战栗，兴奋，害怕

convulsion/kən'vʌlʃn/ n. [医] 惊厥，动乱，震撼，震动

paddy/'pædi/ n. 稻田，水田，稻，稻谷

incidence/'ɪnsɪdəns/ n. 发生率，影响范围

endemic/en'demɪk/ adj. 某地特有的，（尤指疾病）地方性的，风土的

stagnant/'stægnənt/ adj. 不流动的，停滞的，污浊的，不景气的

1.3.6 寨卡病毒病 Zika virus disease

寨卡病毒病是由寨卡病毒引起的蚊媒传染病。世界卫生组织曾在 2016 年 2 月 1 日宣布"小头畸形和其他神经系统疾病聚集性病例"构成"国际关注的突发公共卫生事件"，并指出这些病例与寨卡病毒病流行密切相关。

1. 病原体和临床表现

寨卡病毒病是由寨卡病毒引起的一种病毒性疾病。大部分寨卡病毒感染并没有病征。寨卡病毒感染的病征包括皮疹、发烧、结膜炎、肌肉或关节疼痛和疲累。这些症状一般轻微及持续数天。

Zika virus disease is a mosquito-borne infectious disease caused by Zika virus. On February 1, 2016, the WHO declared "cluster of microcephaly and other neurological disorders" as a "public health emergency of international concern", noting that these cases are closely related to the prevalence of Zika virus disease.

1. Pathogens and clinical features

Zika virus disease is a viral disease caused by Zika virus. Most Zika virus infection is asymptomatic. The symptoms of Zika virus infection include skin rash, fever, conjunctivitis, muscle or joint pain and general malaise. These symptoms are usually mild and last for a few days.

较受关注的是该病对怀孕的不良影响（初生婴儿出现小头畸），以及和其他神经系统及自身免疫性的并发症如格林巴氏综合征的关系。

2. 传播途径

寨卡病毒主要通过受到感染的伊蚊叮咬而传染给人类。它亦在人类精液中被发现，通过性接触传染已被确认，包括男性同性性行为。寨卡病毒亦可能通过其他传播途径，如输血和母婴感染传播。

3. 潜伏期

病症一般于被感染的蚊子叮咬后2~7天出现。

4. 治疗方法

目前并没有治疗寨卡病毒感染的药物，主要是通过症状疗法以舒缓不适及预防脱水。如果病情恶化，患者应立刻就医。

5. 预防方法

现时并没有预防寨卡病毒感染的疫苗。要预防寨卡病毒感染，公众应避免被蚊子叮咬，

The current major concern is its association with adverse pregnancy outcome (microcephaly) and neurological and autoimmune complications such as Guillain-Barre syndrome.

2. Route of transmission

Zika virus is mainly transmitted to humans through the bite of infected Aedes mosquitoes. It has also been found in human semen, and transmission by sexual contact including male homosexual behavior has been confirmed. Other modes of transmission such as blood transfusion and perinatal transmission are possible.

3. Incubation period

Symptoms typically begin 2 to 7 days after the bite of infected mosquitoes.

4. Management

There is no specific medication for Zika virus infection, and the mainstay of treatment is symptomatic relief and prevention of dehydration. If symptoms worsen, patients should seek medical care and advice immediately.

5. Prevention measures

At present, there is no effective vaccine against Zika virus infection. To prevent Zika virus infection, members of the

防止蚊子滋生。

穿着宽松、浅色的长袖上衣及长裤，并于外露的皮肤及衣服涂上含避蚊胺（DEET）成分的昆虫驱避剂。

采取其他户外的预防措施。避免使用有香味的化妆品或护肤品。依照说明重复使用昆虫驱避剂。

外出游客，尤其是有免疫系统疾病或严重长期病患者，于出发前往塞卡病毒持续传播的地区（受影响地区），最少6个星期前咨询医生，并应该采取额外的预防措施，避免受到叮咬。

如到受影响地区的郊外，应带便携式蚊帐并在蚊帐上使用氯菊酯（一种杀虫剂）。切勿将氯菊酯涂在皮肤上。如感到不适，应尽早就医。

外出游客从受影响地区回国后至少21天内须继续使用昆虫驱避剂，若感到身体不适，如发烧，应尽快求医，并将行程细节告知医生。

public are reminded to protect themselves from mosquito bites and prevent mosquito proliferation.

Wear loose, light-colored, long-sleeved tops and trousers, and use DEET-containing insect repellent on exposed parts of the body and clothing.

Take additional preventive measures when going outdoors. Avoid using fragrant cosmetics or skin care products. Re-apply insect repellents according to instructions.

If going to areas with ongoing Zika virus transmission(affected areas), travelers especially persons with immune disorders or severe chronic illnesses, should arrange a consultation with doctor at least 6 weeks before the trip, and take extra preventive measures to avoid mosquito bites.

If travelling in rural affected areas, travelers should carry a portable bed net and apply permethrin (an insecticide) on it. Permethrin should not be applied to skin. Seek medical attention promptly if feeling unwell.

Travelers who return from affected areas should apply insect repellent for at least 21 days after arrival. If feeling unwell, e. g. having fever, travelers should seek medical advice promptly, and provide

孕妇及 6 个月或以上的儿童可以使用含避蚊胺成分的昆虫驱避剂。

Pregnant women and children of 6 months or older can use DEET-containing insect repellent.

Words & Expressions

microcephaly/ˌmaɪkrouˈsefəli/ n. 头小畸型

malaise/məˈleɪz/ n. 不适，不舒服，莫名的不安，萎靡不振

proliferation/prəˌlɪfəˈreɪʃn/ n. 增殖，分芽繁殖，再育，激增

permethrin/pərˈmeθrɪn/ n. 合成除虫菊酯

DEET-containing   含避蚊胺成分

1.4   经体液、血液、血制品传播的疾病
Diseases transmitted by body fluids, blood or blood products

1.4.1   埃博拉病毒病   Ebola virus disease

埃博拉病毒病是由感染埃博拉病毒株引起的一种罕见的和致命的疾病。埃博拉病毒病是严重的、往往致命的人类疾病，病死率高达90%，是世界上最凶猛的疾病之一。埃博拉病毒可以在人类和非人类灵长类动物（猴子和黑猩猩）中发

Ebola virus disease is a rare and deadly disease caused by infection with one of the Ebola virus strains. Ebola virus disease is a severe and often fatal human disease with a high mortality rate of up to 90%. It is one of the most ferocious diseases in the world. Ebola can cause disease in humans and nonhuman primates

病。病情严重的患者需要获得重症支持治疗。在疫情暴发期间，卫生工作者、家庭成员和其他与病人或死者密切接触的人受到感染的风险更高。目前还没有针对埃博拉病毒的有效疫苗或药物。埃博拉病毒感染患者康复产生的抗体持续至少10年。

埃博拉病毒于1976年首次在现刚果民主共和国的埃博拉河附近发现。自那时起，疫情在非洲偶发。1976年6月至2000年10月，埃博拉病毒在非洲苏丹、扎伊尔、加蓬、乌干达四国曾发生过6次大流行。2000年9月，埃博拉在乌干达北部地区古卢暴发，428人感染，224人死亡。

1. 临床表现

感染者症状与感染同为丝状病毒科的马尔堡病毒极为相似，包括恶心、呕吐、肤色改变、全身酸痛、体内出血、腹泻、体外出血、发烧等。死亡率在50%～90%之间，致死原因主要为中风、心肌梗死、低

(monkeys and chimpanzees) . Patients with severe illness need intensive supportive care. During an outbreak, health workers, family members and others who had close contact with the sick or dead are at higher risk of infection. No effective vaccine or medicine is available for Ebola virus in the present. People who recover from Ebola infection develop antibodies that last for at least 10 years.

Ebola virus was first discovered in 1976 near the Ebola River which is now in the Democratic Republic of Congo. Since then, outbreaks have appeared sporadically in Africa. From June 1976 to October 2000, six pandemics occurred in four African countries: Sudan, Zaire, Gabon and Uganda. Ebola struck Gulu in northern Ugandan in September 2000, causing 428 people infected and 224 deaths.

1. Clinical features

The symptoms of infected persons are very similar to Marburg virus in the same family of fibro virology, including nausea, vomiting, skin color change, general soreness, internal bleeding, diarrhea, external bleeding, fever, etc. The mortality rate ranges from 50% to 90%. The main causes of death are stroke, myocardial infarction, hypovolemic

血容量休克或多发性器官衰竭。

2. 潜伏期

可在接触埃博拉病毒后 2～21 天出现症状，平均为8～10天。

3. 传染源

病人是主要的传染源，猴子可能是病毒的自然宿主。

4. 传播途径

直接接触病人的血液、分泌物等体液传播。

通过直接接触病人尸体传播。

处理发病或病死的猩猩、猴等动物引起传播。

医务人员在护理病人时没有采取有效的个人防护也会引起传播。

5. 预防措施

不要处理可能接触过感染者血液或体液的物品。

避免在葬礼上接触埃博拉死亡患者的尸体。

避免接触蝙蝠和非人类灵长类动物或这些动物的血液、液体和生肉。

shock, or multiple organ failure.

2. Incubation period

Symptoms may appear anytime from 2 to 21 days after exposure to Ebola. The incubation period is 8 to 10 days on average.

3. Source of infection

Patients are the main source of infection, and monkeys may be the natural host of the virus.

4. Route of transmission

Direct contact with the patient's blood, secretions, and other body fluids.

Direct contact with dead bodies of sick people.

Dealing with sick or dead orangutans, monkeys, and other animals.

Medical personnel failing to take effective personal protection when caring for patients may also be infected.

5. Prevention measures

Do not handle items that may have come in contact with an infected person's blood or body fluids.

Avoid contact with the body of someone who has died from Ebola on the funeral.

Avoid contact with bats and nonhuman primates or blood, fluids, and raw meat of these animals.

避免前往西非接受埃博拉患者治疗的医院。

要密切注意埃博拉病毒全球疫情动态，加强国境检疫，暂停猴子尤其是来自疫区猴子的进口。

对有出血症状的可疑病人，应隔离观察。一旦确诊应及时报告卫生部门，对病人进行最严格的隔离，即使用带有空气过滤装置的隔离设备。

医护人员、实验人员穿好隔离服，可能时需穿太空服进行检验操作，以防意外。对与病人密切接触者，也应进行密切观察。

Avoid going to hospitals in West Africa where Ebola patients are being treated.

Pay close attention to the epidemic situation of Ebola virus in the world, strengthen frontier quarantine, and suspend the import of monkeys especially from the epidemic areas.

The suspect with bleeding symptoms should be isolated and observed. Once confirmed, the patient should be reported to health authorities in a timely manner, and the patient should be quarantined in the strictest possible, that is, using the isolation equipment with air filtration device.

Medical staff and laboratory staff should wear isolation suits and space suits when possible to conduct inspection operations in case of accidents. Close observation should also be carried out for those who have close contact with patients.

Words & Expressions

Ebola virus　埃博拉病毒

primate/ˈpraɪmeɪt/ n. 灵长目动物（包括人、猴子等），大主教

chimpanzee/ˌtʃɪmpænˈziː/ n. 黑猩猩

orangutan/əˈræŋətæn/ n. 猩猩

infarction/ɪnˈfɑːrkʃn/ n. 梗塞形成，梗死形成

myocardial infarction　心肌梗死

1.4.2 梅毒 Syphilis

梅毒是由梅毒密螺旋体感染而发生的一种性传播疾病，如果没有充分治疗，可能导致长期的并发症或死亡。梅毒在全世界范围内均有分布。

1. 临床表现

感染后 10~90 天出现症状。一期梅毒，出现硬下疳，可能有溃疡；二期梅毒，主要特征是出现皮疹或黏膜损伤（嘴、阴道、肛门等）；晚期梅毒，一期二期梅毒症状消失，进入晚期梅毒，晚期梅毒可能侵袭内脏器官、脑、神经系统、眼睛、心脏、血管、肝脏、骨、关节，还会引起肌肉运动失调、麻痹、失明和痴呆，严重者可致死。

Syphilis is a sexually transmitted disease caused by the bacterium treponema pallidum. Syphilis can cause long-term complications or death if not adequately treated. Syphilis is found throughout the world.

1. Clinical features

The symptoms appear in 10 to 90 days after infection. Primary stage is marked by appearance of a single chancre and there may be ulceration. Secondary stage is marked by skin rashes or mucous membrane lesions(in mouth, vagina, anus, etc.). The late stage begins when primary and secondary symptoms disappear. In the late stage, the disease may damage the internal organs, brain, nerves, eyes, heart, blood vessels, liver, bones and joints. Symptoms of the late stage may also include difficult coordinating muscle movements, paralysis, numbness, gradual blindness, and dementia. This damage may be serious enough to cause death.

2. 潜伏期

潜伏期平均 21 天。

3. 传播途径

梅毒主要通过性接触传播、血液传播和母婴传播（妊娠、生产和哺乳过程传给新生儿）。

4. 预防措施

旅行前，请咨询医生了解目的地该病流行情况及注意事项。

旅行时，杜绝不安全性交等高危行为；不轻易接受输血和血制品（如需使用，要求医院提供经检测合格的血液和血制品）；避免使用患者使用过的餐具、被褥、衣服、毛巾等。

旅行回国入境时或入境后，如出现上述不适，应尽早到医院诊治，并主动告知近期旅行情况（接触史、旅行史等）。

2. Incubation period

The incubation period is 21 days on average.

3. Route of transmission

Syphilis can be transmitted through sexual intercourse, transfusion of contaminated blood and between a mother and her infant during pregnancy, childbirth and breast-feeding.

4. Prevention measures

Consult a doctor about the epidemic situation of the destination before travel.

While traveling, avoid unsafe sexual behaviors, make sure that any blood or blood products you might need are tested for syphilis, and avoid using any quilt, clothes, towel, etc. contaminated by patients of syphilis.

After travel, if any related symptoms develop, see a doctor, and inform him/her of the recent patient contact history, travel history and so on.

Words & Expressions

syphilis/'sɪfɪlɪs/ n. 梅毒

treponema/ˌtrepə'nimə/ n. 密螺旋体

pallidum/'pælɪdəm/ n. 苍白球

chancre/'ʃæŋkər/ n. 下疳，硬下疳

lesion/'liːʒn/ n. 损害，身体器官组织的损伤

numbness/'nʌmnəs/ n. 无感觉，麻木，惊呆

dementia/dɪ'menʃə/ n. ［医］痴呆

treponema pallidum 梅毒密螺旋体，苍白密螺旋体

1.4.3 拉沙热 Lassa fever

拉沙热是由拉沙病毒引起，主要经啮齿类动物传播的一种急性传染病。20 世纪 50 年代首次被发现，但直到 1969 年才分离出病毒。本病主要在几内亚、利比里亚、塞拉利昂和尼日利亚等西非国家流行。据估计，每年新发病例数达 10 万人以上，其中约 1000～3000 人死亡（病死率 1%～3%），住院患者的病死率为 15%～25%。

Lassa fever is an acute infectious disease caused by Lassa virus and transmitted mainly by rodents. It was first identified in the 1950s, but the virus was not isolated until 1969. The disease is endemic mainly in the West African countries such as Guinea, Liberia, Sierra Leone, and Nigeria. It is estimated that there are more than 100,000 new cases per year, of which approximately 1,000 to 3,000 died(1% to 3% of case-fatality rate) and the fatality rate of hospitalized patients is 15% to 25%.

1. 病原体

拉沙病毒属于沙粒病毒科，为负链 RNA 病毒。病毒致病机制目前尚不明确。

2. 临床症状

发热、咳嗽、气短、发冷、咽痛等呼吸道症状和体征，头痛、肌肉痛、关节痛，还有恶心、呕吐、腹泻等胃肠道症状。

3. 潜伏期

拉沙热的潜伏期为 6～12 天，该病通常是渐进性发病，分为三阶段：疲劳、全身无力、发热；头痛、喉咙痛、呕吐、腹泻；面部肿胀，低血压，鼻子出血。

4. 传染源

啮齿动物，拉沙热患者。

5. 传播途径

直接/间接接触老鼠或其排泄物，接触病人或病人血液、尿液或其他分泌物。

6. 预防措施

尚没有疫苗用于预防该病，需要通过如下四方面减少该病

1. Pathogens

Lassa virus is a negative-stranded RNA virus which is belonging to the arenaviruses family. The pathogenesis of the virus is still unclear.

2. Clinical features

Fever, cough, shortness of breath, chills, sore throat and other respiratory symptoms and signs, headache, muscle pain, joint pain, nausea, vomiting, diarrhea, and other gastrointestinal symptoms.

3. Incubation period

The incubation period of Lassa fever is 6 to 12 days. The disease usually develops gradually and can be divided into three stages: fatigue, general weakness and fever; headache, sore throat, vomiting and diarrhea; face swelling, low blood pressure and nose bleeding.

4. Source of infection

Rodents, and Lassa fever patients.

5. Route of transmission

Direct/indirect contact with rats or their excreta, contact with patients or patients' blood, urine, or other secretions.

6. Prevention measures

There is no vaccine to prevent this disease yet. It needs to reduce the

的发生。

控制传染源。加强居室周围生活环境中的灭鼠工作。隔离感染者（疑似及确诊患者），严格处理患者体液和排泄物。迅速和有效开展接触者追踪。

切断传播途径。隔离区内采取呼吸防护措施。在广泛灭鼠的基础上，减少与多乳鼠接触的机会。保护食物及水源免受鼠类污染，保持良好的环境卫生。

保护易感人群。避免接触患者，避免接触鼠类。

与患者密切接触者应使用特定防护用品，如防护服、口罩、手套等。

incidence of the disease in four ways below:

Control the source of infection. Strengthen the control work against rats in the living environment around the house. Isolate the infected (suspected and confirmed) and strictly dispose of the body fluids and excreta of patients. Trace the contacts promptly and effectively.

Cut off transmission routes. Respiratory protection measures should be taken in the isolation area. Reduce the chance of contact with mastomys natalensis. Protect food and water from rodents and maintain good environmental hygiene.

Protect vulnerable groups. Avoid contact with patients and rodents.

People in close contact with the patients should use specific protective equipment, such as protective suits, masks, gloves, etc.

Words & Expressions

strand/strænd/ n. （绳子的）股，绞，串

arenavirus/əˈriːnəvaɪrəs/ n. 沙粒病毒

negative-stranded 负链

mastomys natalensis 多乳鼠类

1.4.4 艾滋病 Acquired immunodeficiency syndrome(AIDS)

艾滋病（AIDS）是获得性免疫缺陷综合征的缩写，是由人类免疫缺陷病毒（HIV）引起的一种病死率很高的严重传染病。目前尚无有效的疫苗和治愈方法，但完全可以防治。

AIDS stands for acquired immunodeficiency syndrome, a severe infectious disease with high death rate, caused by infection with a virus called human immunodeficiency virus（HIV）. There has been no vaccine so far, but still, it is preventable.

1. 临床表现

原发性艾滋病毒感染是艾滋病毒疾病的第一个阶段，病毒首先在体内形成。只有部分人在感染后1~6周可出现发烧、发冷、盗汗、体重减轻、食欲不振等类似病毒性感冒症状，部分感染者身上可能出皮疹，这些表现常在出现后1~4周内自然消失。部分感染者没有经历过"急性感染"，或症状非常轻微，可能没有注意到已感染。

1. Clinical features

Primary HIV infection is the first stage of HIV disease, when the virus first establishes itself in the body. Some people newly infected with HIV（1 to 6 weeks）will experience some "flu-like" symptoms. These symptoms, which usually last for no more than a few days, might include fever, chills, night sweat, weight loss, loss of appetite, and rashes（not cold-like symptoms）, and some of the symptoms may disappear in 1 to 4 weeks after its primary infection. Other people either do not experience "acute infection", or have symptoms so mild that they may not notice them.

未经治疗的感染者一般要经历 2~10 年的潜伏期才会发病。被诊断为艾滋病的患者无普通症状。当免疫系统受损更严重时，才可能有机会感染。病人将会出现不明原因的持续性不规则低烧、慢性腹泻、渐进性消瘦、乏力等，最后死于各种感染性疾病和肿瘤。

艾滋病的临床表现一般具有以下几个特点。

发病以青壮年较多，发病年龄 80%在 18~45 岁，即性生活较活跃的年龄段。

持续广泛性全身淋巴结肿大，特别是颈部、腋窝和腹股沟淋巴结肿大更明显。

并发恶性肿瘤，如卡波西氏肉瘤、淋巴瘤等恶性肿瘤。

中枢神经系统症状，大约 30%的艾滋病病人出现此症状，如头疼、意识障碍等。

It would take 2 to 10 years to full-blown "AIDS" if HIV positive conditions are left with no management. There are no common symptoms for individuals diagnosed with AIDS. When immune system damage is more severe, people may experience opportunistic infections. AIDS patients will suffer from consistent fever, chronic diarrhea, weight loss and fatigue, and consequently die of complex infections or maligned tumors.

The clinical characteristics of AIDS are as follows:

Young adult aged 18 to 45 years old are the vulnerable group, which are active in sex, accounting for 80% of all the HIV positives and AIDS patients.

Extensive lymphadenopathy (swollen lymph nodes), particularly in neck, axilla, and groin.

Some complications like malignant tumors, such as Kaposi's sarcoma and lymphomas.

About 30% of the patients suffer from central-nervous system illness, for instance, severe headache and disturbance of consciousness.

2. 传播途径

已知艾滋病的三种传播途径：

性接触传播：通过感染了艾滋病毒的血液、精液或阴道和宫颈黏膜分泌物（男女或男男之间无保护性的性接触）传播。

血液传播：输入未经检验的血液或血制品传播。

母婴传播：感染了 HIV 的妇女可在妊娠、分娩和哺乳时将病毒传染给孩子。

在日常生活和工作中，与艾滋病病毒感染者或病人握手、拥抱、礼节性接吻、用餐、一起劳动，共用劳动工具、办公用品、钱币、被褥，一起游泳等不传播艾滋病。蚊虫叮咬也不传播艾滋病。

3. 预防方法

了解艾滋病的预防措施，对艾滋病有正确的认识，对于预防艾滋病感染十分必要。

要树立健康的性观念，洁身自爱。如果有不安全性行为，最好每三个月做一次艾滋病

2. Route of transmission

There are three ways in which HIV is known to be transmitted.

Sexual contact transmission: Contact of infected blood, semen, or vaginal and cervical secretions with mucous membranes.

Blood transmission: Injection of infected blood or blood products.

Mother to baby (perinatal) transmission: Transmission from infected mother to fetus, breastfeeding from an infected mother to an infant.

The routine contacts, such as hand-shakings, hugging, kissing, and sharing tools, as well as working with HIV positives in the same office or swimming together could not spread HIV. Mosquito bites cannot spread HIV infections, either.

3. Prevention measures

Awareness of HIV transmission routes and measures for prevention is essential for one to prevent him/her from infection.

One should foster health and sound sexual philosophy and keep the integrity. Should one experience unsafe sex, HIV

毒抗体检测。

尽量减少性伴侣数量，每次性交时全程正确使用质量合格的安全套。

不共用针头、注射器，不共用牙刷、剃须刀或其他可能被血液污染的物品。不用未消毒的器械进行（穿耳、文眉等）医美外科手术。

尽量避免不必要的输血、注射和针刺。需要时，必须要求使用经检验合格的血液及血液制品和经严格消毒的器械、针具。

感染了艾滋病的孕妇可在医生指导下采取医学措施避免胎儿和新生儿感染。

antibody test is necessary at every three months interval to make certainty of previous HIV infection.

The number of sexual partners should be reduced maximally, and whenever one is having sex, he/she should be consistently using a condom with good quality.

Never share needle, or syringe with someone else, and never share toothbrush, shaver or other tools which might be contaminated. It is also necessary to avoid using un-sterilized medical facilities for any surgical operation in beauty saloon or hospital.

Avoid unnecessary blood transfusion and medical injection. Be sure of using sterilized tools or facilities if this transfusion is necessary and inevitable.

Pregnant woman with HIV positive should go through necessary medical procedures under the guidance of medical professionals or doctors in order to avoid fetal and infant infection.

Words & Expressions

immunodeficiency/ˌɪˌmjuːnoʊdɪˈfiʃnsi/ n. 免疫缺陷

malignant/məˈlɪgnənt/ adj. 恶性的，致命的，恶意的，恶毒的

tumor/ˈtuːmər/ n. 瘤

lymphadenopathy/lɪmˌfædəˈnɑːpəθi/ n. 淋巴结病

axilla/ækˈsɪlə/ n. 胳肢窝，腋窝

scarcoma/skɑːˈkoʊmə/ n. 肉瘤

lymphoma/lɪmˈfoʊmə/ n. 淋巴瘤

perinatal/ˌperɪˈneɪtl/ adj. 围产期的，出生前后的

fetus/ˈfiːtəs/ n. 胎，胎儿

syringe/sɪˈrɪndʒ/ n. 注射器，注射筒，灌肠器，注油筒，洗涤器

sterilize/ˈsterəlaɪz/ v. 消毒，使无菌，使失去生育能力，使不起作用

2 旅客通关与健康防护

Customs Clearance and Health Protective Measures

导读：为进一步做好口岸新冠肺炎疫情防控工作，防止疫情经口岸传播，根据《中华人民共和国国境卫生检疫法》及其实施细则等法律法规的规定，海关总署经研究决定，在全国口岸重新启动出入境人员填写《中华人民共和国出/入境健康申明卡》进行健康申报的制度。出入境人员必须向海关卫生检疫部门进行健康申报，并配合做好体温监测、医学巡查、医学排查等卫生检疫工作。

为了自身和他人的健康，旅客应认真如实地填写健康申明卡。真实准确的健康申明信息将有助于海关关员及时了解旅客的健康状况，采取科学有效措施，控制疫情跨境传播。同时，根据《中华人民共和国国境卫生检疫法》《中华人民共和国刑法》的有关规定，如实填报是旅客的一项法律义务，如有隐瞒或虚假填报，造成疫情传播，将依法追究相关责任。为节省出入境时的通关时间，旅客可使用互联网+海关网站、掌上海关或微信小程序，在通关前 24 小时内向海关申报，过关时向海关出示即可。

由于新冠病毒传染性极强，各年龄段人群普遍容易感染。旅客群体具有体量大、流动性强、暴露风险高等特点，是口岸疫情防控的重点人群。同时，旅客应切实加强个人防护意识，了解、掌握相关预防知识，自觉遵守口岸防控政策，积极配合海关部门落实各项措施。

本章不仅包括旅客出境前的"一查二防三申报"、入境须知等通关指引内容，还结合中国疾控中心发布的公众预防提示，对新冠肺炎疫情期间的个人防护和健康提示进行了梳理。

2.1 旅客通关指引 Customs clearance guidelines for passengers

2.1.1 出境须知 Notes for traveling abroad

一是查：出行前要查询相关注意事项。境外旅行首要预防的就是传染病，要提前了解目的地要求，最常遇到的是一些国家对黄热病、霍乱、流行性脑脊髓膜炎疫苗预防接种的要求。最简单有效的方法是向海关或其下属的国际旅行卫生保健中心咨询，还可登录海关总署网站的信息公开专栏查询。一般来说，为保证在旅行前获得有效的免疫保护，所有的疫苗最好在动身前 1 个月完成。如果旅客携带儿童出行，需要注意的是，儿童接种与成人接种是有区别的，应该尽早咨询！

二是防：境外旅行途中要

First, check: Check relevant precautions before traveling abroad. The primary prevention for overseas travel is to know what infectious diseases are possible and know about the destination requirements in advance. The most common ones are the vaccination requirements for yellow fever, cholera and epidemic meningitis. The simplest and most effective way is to consult the customs or its affiliated international travel health care center, or visit the website for the information disclosure column of the General Administration of Customs. In general, to ensure effective immunization protection prior to travel, it is recommended that all vaccinations should be completed one month before departure. If traveling with children, it is important to note that there is a difference between vaccinations for children and vaccinations for adults. Outbound travelers should consult as early as possible!

Second, prevention: During traveling

注意预防传染病，要做好各种健康风险防范，不给病毒、细菌、寄生虫可乘之机。比如，做好个人卫生，一定要勤洗手，谨慎食用生冷食物，拒绝不卫生食品和生水，防止病原菌和寄生虫祸从口入。在人流密集的区域，可以通过佩戴口罩，降低感染呼吸道传染病的风险。去热带、亚热带旅行尤其要注意预防虫媒传染病，做好防蚊防虫措施，避免感染蚊虫传播的登革热、乙型脑炎、疟疾等疾病。尽量不要接触野生动物，比如旱獭、骆驼、蝙蝠、灵长类动物，提防感染鼠疫、埃博拉等烈性传染病。一旦身体有外伤，务必请及时、正确处理伤口！

三是入境健康申报：如果旅客曾经去过传染病疫区，接触过传染病患者，或出现发热、

abroad, travelers should pay attention to the prevention of infectious diseases and all kinds of health risks. Don't give any opportunity for viruses, bacteria or parasites to ruin your trip. For example, do a good job of personal hygiene, wash hands frequently, be cautious with raw and cold food, reject unhygienic food and unboiled water, and prevent pathogenic bacteria and parasites from entering the mouth. The risk of respiratory infections can be reduced by wearing masks in crowded areas. Attention should be paid to the prevention of insect-borne diseases when traveling to tropical and subtropical areas. Mosquito and insect prevention measures should be taken to avoid infection with dengue fever, Japanese encephalitis, malaria and other diseases transmitted by mosquitoes. Avoid contact with wild animals, such as marmots, camels, bats and primates, and watch out for fulminating infectious diseases such as local plagues and Ebola. If you become bit or injured, be sure to treat the wound promptly and correctly!

Third, get a health declaration：If outbound travelers have been to an infectious disease area, or come in contact with an infectious disease patient, or have

咳嗽、呕吐、腹泻、皮疹、肌肉酸痛、浑身无力等症状，请主动、如实向海关人员申报。这些信息非常重要，能让经验丰富的海关人员快速完成流行病学调查，并通过医学排查和其他必要的方法确定旅客的健康状况，让旅客在最短的时间内得到医疗救助，避免引发可能的公共安全事件！

symptoms such as a fever, cough, vomiting, diarrhea, rash, muscle pain, or experience general weakness, please report to the customs officers actively and truthfully. This information is very important to enable experienced customs officers to quickly complete epidemiological investigations and determine travelers' health status through medical screening and other necessary methods, so that travelers can receive medical assistance in the shortest possible time and avoid any possible public safety incidents!

做好"一查二防三申报"，健康旅行才能没烦恼。一些传染病有潜伏期，旅客入境之后要继续关注自身状况，发现异常请及时就医。

Know about "First Check, Second Prevention and Third Declaration" in advance. It will create a great peace of mind for a healthy travel. Some infectious diseases have an incubation period. Travelers should continue to pay attention to health conditions after entry, and see a doctor right away if travelers notice any abnormalities in body.

2.1.2 入境须知 Notes for entering a country

旅客到达机场或口岸后，可通过填写纸质版本或通过"海关旅客指尖服务小程序"

After arriving at an airport or port, inbound travelers can make a declaration by filling out the paper form or on the Wechat

进行申报，应将健康申明卡主动提交给海关关员，并配合海关做好卫生检疫工作。如旅客有发热、乏力、干咳、呼吸困难等不适症状，应及时与海关关员联系。

1. 入境前

来华和在华的外籍人员需要提前了解入境要求、发病处理方法、就诊方式、日常注意事项，以免无法入境。

入境前请填写健康申明卡。

外籍人士来华后与中国公民采取相同的疫情防控措施。

2. 入境时

旅客在入境时如有下列情况，请立即告知身边的工作人员：

如果入境旅客 14 天内去过新冠肺炎疫情严重的国家和地区，请立即告诉附近的工作人员。

"Customs Passenger Fingertip Service Applet". Travelers should submit the health declaration card to the customs officers actively and cooperate with them for health quarantine. If inbound travelers are showing such symptoms as fever, fatigue, dry cough, difficulty breathing, etc., please contact the customs officers immediately.

1. Before entry

Foreigners coming to and being in China need to know about the entry requirements, measures to handle the onset of disease, ways to get treatment and daily precautions in advance to avoid denial of entry.

Fill in the health declaration card before entry.

Foreigners in China should take the same prevention and control measures as the Chinese citizens do.

2. Entering the country

If a passenger has conditions below, please inform nearby staff members immediately:

If you have been to any country or region where COVID-19 epidemic was severe in the past 14 days, please inform the staff nearby immediately.

如果旅客 14 天内与新冠肺炎病人接触过，请立即告知身边的工作人员。

来自新冠肺炎疫情高发地区的人员可能会被集中隔离进行医学观察。

新冠肺炎病人的密切接触者将被集中隔离进行医学观察。

如果旅客乘坐的交通工具中出现发热病人，可能将被集中隔离进行医学观察。

如果旅客正在发烧并且咳嗽、呼吸困难，请立即告诉附近的工作人员。需要时请拨打 120 急救电话。

如果旅客有发烧、咳嗽、乏力的症状，请一定尽快去医院的发热门诊看病，以免造成严重后果。去医院发热门诊可以拨打 120 急救电话。

如果旅客不幸确诊了新冠肺炎，会被送到指定的医院治疗。工作人员可能会了解旅客的基本信息、联系方式、健康状况、最近去过的地方、最近接触过的人员等情况，请一定要配合。

If you have been in contact with a COVID-19 patient in the past 14 days, please inform the staff nearby immediately.

Travelers coming from areas with a high incidence of COVID-19 may be put in quarantine for medical observation.

Travelers who have had close contact with COVID-19 patients will be put in quarantine for medical observation.

If you have taken the same vehicle with a feverish patient, you may be put in quarantine for medical observation.

If you have a fever, cough or difficulty in breathing, please inform the staff nearby immediately. If necessary, please dial the emergency number 120.

If you have a fever, cough, and fatigue, please go to the fever clinic of a hospital as soon as possible to avoid serious consequences. You can dial the emergency number 120 to ask for an ambulance.

If you are diagnosed with COVID-19, you will be sent to a designated hospital for treatment. Please cooperate with the staff when you are asked for basic personal information, such as your phone number, your health status, places you've been to and people you've had contact with recently.

2.1.3 如何做好健康申报 How to make a health declaration

为有效防范新冠肺炎疫情传播，保护出入境旅客的健康，根据《中华人民共和国国境卫生检疫法》，请旅客按照中国海关要求，认真、如实填写健康申明卡，申报其健康情况和旅行经历。如曾在过去14天途经或停留过新冠肺炎疫情高发国家、地区，或目前有发热、乏力、干咳、呼吸困难等症状，请尽早如实向海关报告。也可通过填写纸质版本或"海关旅客指尖服务小程序"进行申报。抵达后，请将健康申明卡主动提交给海关关员，配合海关做好卫生检疫工作。

出入境人员在出入境时应主动向海关申报，配合海关关员做好体温监测、医学巡查等卫生检疫工作。如实填报健康申明卡是出入境人员必须履行

To effectively contain the spread of COVID-19 and protect the health of inbound and outbound travelers, according to the Frontier Health and Quarantine Law of the People's Republic of China, please fill out the Exit/Entry Health Declaration Form to declare health conditions and travel history truthfully. If travelers have been to, either for a visit or transit, any hard-hit countries or regions during the past 14 days, or if travelers are showing such symptoms as fever, fatigue, dry cough, difficulty breathing, etc. , please report to the customs officers immediately. Travelers can also complete health declaration by hand writing or on the WeChat "Customs Passenger Fingertip Service Applet". When arriving, please give the Health Declaration Form to customs officers, and cooperate with them in health quarantine procedures.

When passing the borders, inbound and outbound travelers must declare to customs officers proactively and cooperate with them on temperature monitoring, medical screening, and other health quarantine

的法律义务。根据《中华人民共和国刑法》第三百三十二条第一款的有关规定，如有隐瞒或虚假填报，造成疫情传播或有传播严重危险的，将可能被处以三年以下有期徒刑或者拘役等刑事处罚。

measures. It is the obligation for international travelers to fill out the Health Declaration Form truthfully. According to Article 332 of the Criminal Law of the People's Republic of China, anyone who conceals or falsely declares the information, causing the spread of quarantinable communicable diseases or a serious danger of spreading them, shall be sentenced to not more than three years of fixed-term imprisonment, criminal detention or other criminal punishment.

2.2　健康防护措施　Health protective measures

2.2.1　减少外出活动　Reducing outdoor activities

避免去疾病正在流行的地区。

建议疫情防控期间减少走亲访友和聚餐，尽量在家休息。

减少到人员密集的公共场所活动，尤其是空气流动性差的地方，例如公共浴池、温泉、影院、网吧、KTV、商场、车站、机场、码头、展览馆等。

Avoid visiting areas where the disease is prevalent.

It is recommended to make less visits to relatives and friends and dining together during the epidemic prevention and control, and stay at home as much as possible.

Try to avoid visits to crowded public areas, especially places of poor ventilation, such as public bathrooms, hot springs, cinemas, internet bars, Karaokes, shopping malls, bus/train stations, airports, ferry terminals and exhibition centers, etc.

2.2.2 个人防护和手卫生 Personal protection and hand hygiene

建议外出佩戴口罩。外出前往公共场所、就医和乘坐公共交通工具时，佩戴医用外科口罩或 N95 口罩。

保持手卫生。减少接触公共场所的公共物品和部位；从公共场所返回、咳嗽手捂之后、饭前便后，用洗手液或香皂流水洗手，或者使用含酒精成分的免洗洗手液；不确定手是否清洁时，避免用手接触口鼻眼；打喷嚏或咳嗽时，用衣肘遮住口鼻。

It is recommended that a mask shall be worn when going out. A surgical or N95 mask shall be worn when visiting public areas, hospitals or taking public transportation.

Keep hands sanitized. Try to avoid touching public objects and parts in public areas. After returning from public areas, coughing with hands to cover the mouth, using the restroom, and before meals, wash your hands with soap or liquid soap under running water, or use alcoholic hand sanitizer. Avoid touching your mouth, nose or eyes when you are unsure whether your hands are clean or not. Cover your mouth and nose with your elbow when you sneeze or cough.

2.2.3 健康监测和就医 Health monitoring and seeking medical attention

------

主动做好个人与家庭成员的健康监测，自觉发热时要主动测量体温。家中有小孩的，要早晚摸小孩的额头，如有发热要为其测量体温。

Monitor the health conditions of your family members and yourself. Measure your temperatures when you feel like having a fever. If you have kid(s) at home, touch the kid's forehead in the morning and at night.

若出现可疑症状，应主动戴上口罩及时就近就医。若出现新冠病毒感染可疑症状（包括发热、咳嗽、咽痛、胸闷、呼吸困难、轻度纳差、乏力、精神稍差、恶心呕吐、腹泻、头痛、心慌、结膜炎、四肢或腰背部肌肉轻度酸痛等），应根据病情，及时到医疗机构就诊。

尽量避免乘坐地铁、公共汽车等交通工具，避免前往人群密集的场所。就诊时应主动告诉医生自己的相关疾病流行地区的旅行居住史，以及发病后接触过什么人，配合医生开展相关调查。

Measure the kid's temperature in case of fever.

Wear a mask and seek medical attention at nearby hospitals in case of suspicious symptoms. Go to medical institution in a timely manner in case the suspicious symptoms relating to the pneumonia caused by novel coronavirus are found. Such symptoms include fever, cough, pharyngalgia, chest distress, dyspnea, mildly poor appetite, feebleness, mild lethargy, nausea, diarrhea, headache, palpitation, conjunctivitis, mildly sore limb or back muscles, etc.

Try to avoid taking metro, bus and other public transportation and visiting crowded areas. Tell the doctor your travel and residence history in epidemic areas, and who you met after you got the disease. Cooperate with your doctor on the relevant queries.

2.2.4 保持良好卫生和健康习惯 Keeping good hygiene and health habits

居室勤开窗，经常通风。

家庭成员不共用毛巾，保持家居、餐具清洁，勤晒衣被。

Frequently open the windows of your house for better ventilation.

Do not share towels with your family members. Keep your home and tableware clean. Sun-cure your clothes and quilts often.

不随地吐痰，口鼻分泌物用纸巾包好，弃置于有盖垃圾箱内。

Do not spit. Wrap your oral and nasal secretion with tissue and throw it in a covered dustbin.

注意营养，适度运动。

Balance your nutrition and exercise moderately.

不要接触、购买和食用野生动物；尽量避免前往售卖活体动物的市场。

Do not touch, buy or eat wild animals. Try to avoid visiting markets that sell live animals.

家庭备置体温计、医用外科口罩或 N95 口罩、家用消毒用品等物资。

Prepare thermometer, surgical or N95 masks, domestic disinfectant and other supplies at home.

2.2.5　健康防护常用表达　Useful expressions for health protection

避免去疾病正在流行的地区，定期用酒精擦手或用肥皂水彻底清洗双手。经常用流水认真洗手，洗手时要使用肥皂或洗手液。没有洗手时，不要用手触碰嘴、鼻子、眼睛。用手接触他人、触摸动物、触碰别人碰过的公共物品后，要及时洗手。

Avoid visiting areas where the disease is prevalent. Regularly and thoroughly clean your hands with an alcohol-based hand rub or wash them with soap and water. Wash your hands often and carefully with running water and soap or hand sanitizer. Avoid touching your mouth, nose or eyes with your unwashed hands. Wash hands in time after touching other people, animals or items for public use.

打喷嚏或咳嗽时，要用纸巾或胳膊遮挡口鼻，不要用手

Cover your mouth and nose with facial tissue or your elbow instead of your hands

遮挡口鼻。

要经常开窗通风，保持室内清洁。

外出回来后，换下外衣、外裤和鞋子。及时清洁手机等常用随身物品。

减少不必要的外出。外出时要戴口罩，最好戴医用口罩。摘下口罩时不要触碰口罩的内外两侧。

尽量减少触摸公共场所的公共物品，例如楼梯扶手、门把手、公用电话等。

尽量减少到人员密集或空气不流通的场所，例如车站、机场、码头、商场、医院、公共卫生间等。如果必须到人员密集或空气不流通的场所，要戴口罩，减少停留时间，与他人保持一定距离。

尽量减少乘坐公共交通工具。如果必须乘坐公共交通工具，要戴口罩，开窗通风，与他人保持一定距离。

尽量减少在公共餐厅就餐。如果必须在公共餐厅就餐，要缩短就餐时间，与其他人保持一定距离。

when you sneeze or cough.

Open windows frequently for air flow and keep the room clean.

Take off your coat, trousers and shoes, and clean your personal belongings such as smart phones upon arriving home.

Avoid going out unless necessary. Wear a mask when going out, preferably a medical mask. Avoid touching both sides of the mask when taking it off.

Try not to touch items in public places such as handrails, door handles, public telephones and so on.

Try not to visit places with crowds or poor ventilation, such as railway stations, airports, ship terminals, shopping malls, hospitals, public toilets and so on. If you have to visit places with crowds or poor ventilation, wear a mask, stay shorter, and keep a distance from others.

Try not to take public transportation. If you have to take public transportation, wear a mask, open the windows, and keep a distance from others.

Try not to have meals in restaurants. If you have to eat in a restaurant, try to eat quickly and keep a distance from others.

不要在人多时乘坐电梯，不要用手直接接触电梯按钮，尽量走楼梯。

尽量使用非接触的打招呼方式，减少握手、拥抱、亲吻等接触式社交礼仪。

经常测量体温，了解自己的健康情况。

如果自己出现发烧、干咳的症状，且近期去过疫情发生地或者身边有新冠肺炎患者，要尽快联系当地医疗机构或专业管理机构。

如果怀疑自己被传染，要尽快咨询当地医疗机构或专业管理机构。

如果身边有人发烧、咳嗽、浑身乏力，要与其保持安全距离，并提醒其及时去看病。

要特别注意儿童、老人、残障人士在学校、幼儿园、养老院、社会福利机构等场所的疫情防护情况。

要饮食均衡，适当运动，作息规律，避免过度疲劳。

要从权威渠道了解疫情信

Do not take a crowded elevator or push buttons with your hands directly. Try to take the stairs.

Greet others without touching them, and reduce contact social etiquette like handshake, hug or kiss.

Take your temperature often to track your health condition.

If you have a fever and dry cough, and recently visited a COVID-19-hit place or had close contact with COVID-19 patients, please contact local medical units or professional control institutions immediately.

If you suspect that you are infected, please seek advice from local medical units or professional control institutions at once.

If you find people with fever, cough and fatigue around you, keep a safe distance from them and advise them to see a doctor.

Give special protection to children, the elderly and the disabled against COVID-19 epidemic in schools, kindergartens, nursing homes and other social welfare places.

Have a balanced diet, take proper exercise, get regular rest and avoid over fatigue.

Get COVID-19 information via

息，做好科学防护，保持良好心态，不要恐慌。

authoritative channels, take effective protections, keep a good mood and avoid panic.

Words & Expressions

trauma/ˈtrɔːmə/ n. 创伤，损伤，痛苦经历，挫折

marmot/ˈmɑːrmət/ n. 旱獭，土拨鼠

applet/ˈæplət/ n. 支程序，小应用程序，小型程式，程序类型

feebleness/ˈfiːblnəs/ n. 弱，微弱

lethargy/ˈleθərdʒi/ n. 昏睡，没精打采，懒洋洋，嗜眠症

palpitation/ˌpælpəˈteʃən/ n. 心悸

disclosure column　公开专栏

quarantinable communicable diseases　检疫传染病

3 口岸卫生检疫场景表达

Dialogues in Scenes of Health Quarantine at Ports

导读：旅客出入境时，须接受卫生检疫。海关对出入境人员采取健康申报、体温监测和医学巡查等检疫方式。一旦发现有传染病症状的人员，立即安排其进入（负压）检疫排查室进行流行病学调查和医学排查。在重大烈性传染病疫情防控期间，海关可对重点人群采取专区查验的方式，并有权要求出入境人员如实填写健康申明卡，出示某种传染病的预防接种证书、健康证明或者其他有关证件。

对有传染病症状的人员，应首先进行包括体温复测、流行病学调查以及医学检查等内容的排查，并做出初步判断。初步判定排除传染病感染嫌疑的，登记个人信息，给予健康建议，发放就诊方便卡放行。无法排除传染病感染嫌疑的，经当事人知情同意，可采集样本送实验室检测。无法排除检疫传染病染疫嫌疑的，或在重大疫情防控期间征得本人同意后，可将其转运至医院进行（隔离）诊治。实验室对样品进行病原体检测。

疫苗被寄予了战胜新冠肺炎疫情的厚望，目前已开始在世界各地广泛接种。接种新冠疫苗是保护人群并遏制病毒传播最经济、最有效的手段之一，能有效降低重症和死亡的发生。接种疫苗能够对个体进行有效保护，也对人群进行有效保护，形成健康免疫屏障，这是世界各国（地区）当前防控新冠肺炎疫情最主要的策略之一。

本章内容主要包括口岸卫生检疫场景表达，根据防疫需要，还增加了接种疫苗的场景表达。

3.1 健康申报 Health declaration

1. 请您将出/入境健康申明卡交给我，如您尚未填报，请现场填写。您可以选择填写纸质版本或通过微信小程序进行填报。

2. 根据《中华人民共和国国境卫生检疫法》及其实施细则要求，海关有权要求进出境人员如实逐项填报出/入境健康申明卡，联系方式和住址务必详细准确填写，如有隐瞒或虚假填报，将依法追究相关责任。

3. （如发现填报项目不全或不符合要求）旅客您好！您的出/入境健康申明卡这些项目填写不全/不符合要求，请补充/修改填报。

4. （如发现申报疾病症状或具有防控方案中流行病学史）旅客您好！由于您申报了有关症状/流行病学史，为了保护您和他人的健康，我们将对

1. Sir/Madam, please give me your Exit/Entry Health Declaration Form. If you haven't filled it out yet, you can do it now, either by hand writing or on the WeChat applet.

2. According to the Frontier Health and Quarantine Law of the People's Republic of China and its implementation rules, you are required to fill out the Exit/Entry Health Declaration Form truthfully. In particular, please make sure that your contact number and address information is specific and correct. If you conceal or falsely declare the information, you will be held accountable according to the law.

3. Sir/Madam, your Exit/Entry Health Declaration Form is not complete/doesn't meet the requirements. Please add information/revise the information again.

4. Sir/Madam, because you have declared relevant symptoms/ a history of infectious disease, for your health and that of others, we will need to ask you some questions and do some medical examination.

您进行有关询问和排查，请您理解和配合。

Thank you for your understanding and cooperation.

3.2 医学巡查 Initial health assessment

1. 旅客您好！我们观察到您的体态/面容有异常，请问您是否有发热、咳嗽、乏力、腹泻等不适症状？

2.（如当事人确认有不适症状）为了您和他人的健康，请您戴上口罩和手套，随我到医学排查室进行健康检查。

1. Sir/Madam, your body/face doesn't look well. Do you have symptoms like fever, cough, fatigue（feeling tired）, or diarrhea, etc. ?

2. For the health of you and others, please put on the face mask and gloves, and follow me to the medical examination room.

3.3 体温监测 Temperature monitoring

1. 旅客您好！经红外体温监测，您的体温超过了37℃，我们需要对您进行体温复测，请问您是否有发热、咳嗽、乏力、腹泻等不适症状？

2. 请将体温计放在腋（腋窝）下夹紧。测温需要5分钟。

3. 时间到了，请将体温计取出来给我。

4.（如当事人体温复测超

1. Sir/Madam, the infrared thermometer shows that your body temperature is above 37 degrees Celsius. We have to take your temperature again. Do you have symptoms such as fever, cough, fatigue（feeling tired）, or diarrhea, etc. ?

2. Please clamp the thermometer under your arm（armpit）. It will take 5 minutes.

3. Time's up. Let me check your temperature.

4. Your temperature is 39 degrees

过 37.3℃）您的体温是 39℃，您发烧了。

5. 为了您和他人的健康，请您戴上口罩和手套，随我到医学排查室进行健康检查。

Celsius. You have a fever.

5. For the health of you and others, please put on the face mask and gloves, and follow me to the medical examination room.

3.4 流行病学调查 Epidemiological investigation

1. 旅客您好！由于您具有相关疾病症状，为了您和他人的健康，根据《中华人民共和国国境卫生检疫法》及其实施细则要求，我们需要对您进行流行病学调查，请您配合并如实回答。

2. 请问过去 14 日内您在中国（包含港澳台地区）旅行或居住过吗？如有，请列明具体的城市。

3. 如果您在过去 14 天内访问过别的国家和地区，请列明。

4. 过去 14 日内，您曾接触过新冠肺炎确诊病例/疑似病例/无症状感染者吗？

5. 过去 14 日内，您曾接

1. Sir/Madam, since you are showing certain disease symptoms, for the health of you and others, we have to conduct an epidemiological investigation on you according to the Frontier Health and Quarantine Law of the People's Republic of China and its implementation rules. Please cooperate with us and answer our questions truthfully.

2. Have you visited/lived in China during the past 14 days, including Hong Kong, Macao and Taiwan regions? If yes, please list the cities you have visited.

3. If you have visited other countries and regions during the past 14 days, please specify.

4. Have you had direct contact with confirmed/suspected/symptomless cases of COVID-19 during the past 14 days?

5. Have you had direct contact with

触过发热和/或有呼吸道症状的患者吗?

6. 过去 14 日内,您所居住社区曾报告有新冠肺炎病例吗?

7. 过去 14 日内,您所在的办公室/家庭是否出现 2 人及以上有发热和/或呼吸道症状?

8. 现在或过去 14 日内,您是否有以下症状?包括发热、寒颤、干咳、咳痰、鼻塞、流涕、咽痛、头痛、乏力、头晕、肌肉酸痛、关节酸痛、气促、呼吸困难、胸闷、胸痛、结膜充血、恶心、呕吐、腹泻、腹痛或其他症状。

9. 过去 14 日内,您是否曾服用退烧药、感冒药或止咳药?

10. 过去 14 日内,您曾接受过新冠病毒检测吗?检测结果是阳性还是阴性?

people having fever and/or symptoms of respiratory infection during the past 14 days?

6. Has your community reported any COVID-19 case during the past 14 days?

7. Have there been two or more members in your office/family who got fever and/or had symptoms of respiratory infection during the past 14 days?

8. Do you have now, or have you had in the past 14 days, the following symptoms? Including fever, chills, dry cough, expectoration, stuffy nose, running nose, sore throat, headache, fatigue, dizziness, muscle pain, arthralgia, shortness of breath, breathing difficulty, chest tightness, chest pain, conjunctival congestion, nausea, vomiting, diarrhea, stomachache, or other symptoms.

9. Have you taken any medication for fever, cold or cough during the past 14 days?

10. Have you been tested for COVID-19 during the past 14 days? Is the result positive or negative?

3.5 医学排查 Medical examination

1. 旅客您好！经过对您的流行病学调查，我们目前无法排除您的传染病感染嫌疑。为进一步确定，我们需要对您进行有关医学排查，请您配合。

2. 旅客您好！为进一步确定您是否可能感染传染病，我们需要对您进行鼻咽拭子/咽拭子/痰液和血样采集，请您配合。

3. 如果您同意采样，请在这份文件上签名。

4.（采集咽拭子）请张开嘴，"啊"出声。

5.（采集痰液）请咳深部痰液，不要吐口水。请将痰液吐到无菌杯中。

6.（采集血液）您有晕针、晕血史吗？请您做几次握紧、松开拳头好吗？请按压三分钟。

7. 请您放松，很快就会好的。

1. Sir/Madam, according to the result of your epidemiological investigation, we can't rule out the possibility of infection. Therefore, a medical examination is necessary. Thank you for your cooperation.

2. Sir/Madam, we have to collect a nasopharyngeal swab specimen/ throat swab specimen/ sputum sample and blood sample in order to further determine whether you are infected with any infectious disease. Thank you for your cooperation.

3. If you agree, please sign here.

4. Open your mouth and say "ah".

5. Please cough up the sputum from the deep throat. Don't spit dribbles. Spit the sputum to the sample cup.

6. Have you fainted at the sight of needles or blood? Could you clench and unclench your fist a few times please? Please press for 3 minutes.

7. Relax, please. It'll be all right soon.

3.6　转诊处置　Transfer for treatment

旅客您好！经过对您的流行病学调查和医学排查，结合您的血常规检测情况，目前无法排除您的传染病感染嫌疑。按照《中华人民共和国国境卫生检疫法》及其实施细则要求，为了您和他人的健康，我们将通过急救车，将您转运至指定医院进一步诊治。救护车会尽快到来，请您耐心等待。

Sir/Madam, according to the results of your epidemiological investigation, medical examination and blood test, the possibility of infection can't be ruled out. Therefore, according to the Frontier Health and Quarantine Law of the People's Republic of China and its implementation rules, for your health and that of others, you are going to be transferred to the designated hospital by ambulance for further diagnosis. The ambulance will be here soon. Please wait here. Thank you.

3.7　接种疫苗　Vaccination

疫苗接种能产生免疫力，是预防性地保护人群、遏制病毒传播经济且有效的手段。

1. 请在你的预约时间之前10分钟到达。

2. 到达之后，你会被问及一系列的筛查问题。

3. 如果你感到不适，或者是有新冠肺炎症状，不要来接

Vaccination can produce immunity, which is an economical and effective way to protect the population groups prophylactically and to contain the spread of the virus.

1. Please arrive 10 minutes before your scheduled appointment time.

2. When you arrive, you will be asked a series of screening questions.

3. If you are unwell or have symptoms of COVID-19, you are not allowed to come

种中心。

4. 请带好医疗卡，还有政府颁发的身份证明或居住证明。

5. 通过筛查之后，你需要签到，并且同意打疫苗。

6. 接种疫苗。

7. 接种后等候 30 分钟。

对话一

A：你的预约是几点的？

B：下午 3:45。

A：我们现在在做下午3:30那一组。你有点早了，所以请排队等候。

B：好的。

A：我需要问你几个问题。你在过去 14 天内出过国吗？

B：没有。

A：你有没有和已经确诊新冠肺炎或是可能确诊的病人有过密切接触？

B：没有。

A：你有没有被要求自我隔离？

B：没有。

A：好的，你可以进去了。

to the vaccination centre.

4. Please bring your health card, another identification or residency proof issued by the government.

5. After passing the screening process, you will be asked to check in and agree to the vaccination.

6. Get vaccinated.

7. Wait 30 minutes after vaccination.

Dialogue 1

A：What time is your appointment?

B: It's 3: 45pm.

A: We are now dealing with the appointment of 3: 30pm. You are a bit early. So, please wait in the line.

B: OK.

A：I'm just gonna ask you a few questions. Have you been abroad in the past 14 days?

B: No.

A：Have you been in close contact with someone who was or might have been diagnosed with COVID-19?

B: No.

A：Have you been asked to isolate yourself?

B: No.

A: OK. You can get inside now.

请消毒手，摘下口罩，再次消毒手。请戴上这个新的口罩。你现在可以去注册柜台了。

B：好的。

A：请给我你的医疗卡。你还住在 42 街吗？

B：是的。

A：都办好了。请走到走廊的尽头，然后左转。

B：谢谢。

对话二

A：你今天打的是辉瑞/科兴新冠肺炎疫苗。你有什么过敏吗？

B：没有。

A：这是你的第一针。

B：好的。

A：你用哪只手写字？

B：我用右手。

A：好，我打到你的左边胳膊上。请把你的袖子卷起来。

B：好的。

A：打好了。你会感觉胳膊上有刺痛，就像被蚊子叮咬一样。你明天可能感觉胳膊有些疼痛，也有可能会肿起来。你

Sanitize your hands please. Take off your mask. Sanitize your hands again. Put on this new mask please. Now you can go to the check-in desk.

B: OK.

A：Can I have your health card please? Are you still living at Street No. 42?

B: Yes.

A: You are all set now. Go to the end of the hall and turn left.

B: Thanks.

Dialogue 2

A：So, you are getting the Pfizer/Sinovac COVID-19 vaccine today. Do you have any allergy?

B: No.

A: This is your first dose.

B: OK.

A：Which hand do you use to write?

B: I use my right hand.

A: OK, I will give you an injection in your left arm then. Could you roll up your sleeve please?

B: OK.

A: You are done. You will feel a sting on your arm. It's like a mosquito bite. You might feel some pain in your arm tomorrow. It might be swollen too. You can take an

可以用冰敷，或者吃止疼药。

B：好的。

A：100 万接种人员里面可能会有一个人有荨麻疹、面部肿大或呼吸困难等症状。如果是这样的话，你可以马上打120。你还有什么问题吗？

B：没了，都挺好的。

A：这是你的接种卡。你会收到邮件通知你打第二针的。你可以去休息区了。

B：谢谢。

ice compress or take a pain killer.

B: OK.

A：One in a million of people will develop symptoms such as hives, swelling of the face or breathing difficulties. If that's the case, you can call 120 immediately. Do you have any questions?

B: No. I'm good.

A: This is your "Vaccination Card". You will receive an e-mail for the second dose. You can proceed to the resting area now.

B: Thank you.

Words & Expressions

infrared/ˌɪnfrəˈred/ adj. ［物］红外线的

Celsius/ˈselsiəs/ n. 摄氏度；adj. 摄氏的

expectoration/ɪkˌspektəˈreɪʃn/ n. 咳痰

pharyngeal/fəˈrɪndʒiəl/ adj. 咽的，咽音，咽部；n. 咽音

swab/swɑːb/ n. （医用的）拭子，药签，（用拭子取下的）化验样本；v. 用拭子拭抹或擦净（某物），（用拖把、抹布等）擦洗（某物）

sputum/ˈspjuːtəm/ n. 痰

vaccinate/ˈvæksɪneɪt/ v. 接种疫苗（多用被动），给……接种疫苗，注射疫苗

jab/dʒæb/ n. 接种（＝injection）；v. 戳，刺

prophylactic/ˌproʊfəˈlæktɪk/ adj. 预防（性）的；n. 预防剂，预防用品

prophylactically/ˌproʊfəˈlæktɪkli/ adv. ［医］预防地，预防上

screen/skriːn/ n. 屏幕，掩蔽物，纱门；v. 放映，遮挡，检查，筛选

proof/pruːf/ n. 证明，检验，证据

residency/ˈrezɪdənsi/ n. 住所

allergy/ˈælərdʒi/ n. 过敏反应，厌恶，反感

sting/stɪŋ/ v. 叮，螫，刺痛，刺激；n. 螫伤处，（某些昆虫的）毒刺，（身体或心灵的）剧痛

hives/haɪvz/ n. [医] 荨麻疹，蜂箱（hive 的名词复数），蜂巢，喧闹地区

the infrared thermometer　红外测温仪

nasopharyngeal swab　鼻咽拭子

throat swab　咽拭子

be vaccinated＝get the jab　接种疫苗

get vaccinated　打疫苗

get the COVID-19 jab　接种新冠肺炎疫苗

self-isolation　自我隔离

all set　都（准备）好了

roll up　卷起来

4 口岸卫生检疫相关规范文件
Related Standard Documents for Health Quarantine at Ports

导读：中国海关进行卫生检疫的执法依据主要有：《国际卫生条例 (2005)》、《中华人民共和国国境卫生检疫法》及其实施细则、《中华人民共和国出境入境管理法》、《中华人民共和国传染病防治法》、《海关总署关于重新启动出入境人员填写健康申明卡制度的公告》等。

《国际卫生条例（2005）》要求各缔约方应当发展、加强和保持其快速有效应对国际关注的突发公共卫生事件的应急核心能力。中国作为世界卫生组织的成员，海关作为《国际卫生条例（2005）》的口岸卫生当局，负有履行《国际卫生条例》的职责与义务。

《中华人民共和国国境卫生检疫法》及其实施细则主要明确了卫生检疫的目的、职责、机构、检疫对象、实施方法及法律责任。卫生检疫的工作内容包括检疫查验、传染病监测、卫生监督、卫生处理、突发公共卫生事件的应对以及核心能力建设等方面，检疫对象涵盖出入境交通工具、人员、货物、行李等。

《中华人民共和国出境入境管理法》明确"禁止外国人入境的疾病"包括严重精神障碍、传染性肺结核病或者有可能对公共卫生造成重大危害的其他传染病。

《中华人民共和国传染病防治法》将我国发病率较高、流行面较大的 41 种传染病列为法定管理传染病，分为甲、乙、丙三类以及埃博拉病毒病，实行分类管理①。新冠肺炎已经被纳入《中华人民共和国传染病防治法》规定的乙类传染病，按甲类传染病管理。

本章摘录了口岸卫生检疫涉及的有关法规制度，方便出入境旅客知悉和海关关员掌握。

---

① 甲类传染病包括：鼠疫、霍乱。乙类传染病包括：传染性非典型肺炎、艾滋病、病毒性肝炎、脊髓灰质炎、人感染高致病性禽流感、麻疹、流行性出血热、狂犬病、流行性乙型脑炎、登革热、炭疽、细菌性和阿米巴性痢疾、肺结核、伤寒和副伤寒、流行性脑脊髓膜炎、百日咳、白喉、新生儿破伤风、梅毒、疟疾等。丙类传染病包括：流行性感冒、流行性腮腺炎、风疹、急性出血性结膜炎等。

4.1 卫生检疫涉及的法规制度
Laws and regulations concerning health quarantine

4.1.1 填写健康申明卡的法律依据
Legal basis for filling out the Exit/Entry Health Declaration Form

1. 关于重新启动出入境人员填写健康申明卡制度的公告

为进一步做好口岸新型冠状病毒感染的肺炎疫情防控工作，防止疫情经口岸传播，根据《中华人民共和国国境卫生检疫法》及其实施细则等法律法规的规定，海关总署经研究决定在全国口岸重新启动出入境人员填写《中华人民共和国出/入境健康申明卡》进行健康申报的制度。出入境人员必须向海关卫生检疫部门进行健康申报，并配合做好体温监测、医学巡查、医学排查等卫生检疫工作。

1. Announcement on Restarting the System of Filling out the Health Declaration Form for Personnel Entering and Exiting China

In order to further effectively conduct the prevention and control of the novel coronavirus pneumonia epidemic at ports and prevent the spread of the epidemic through ports, in accordance with the provisions of the Frontier Health and Quarantine Law of the People's Republic of China and the detailed rules for the implementation thereof, and other relevant laws and regulations, the General Administration of Customs has decided upon deliberation to restart the system of filling out the Health Declaration Form of the People's Republic of China for Personnel Entering and Exiting China at all ports of China for health declaration. The personnel entering and exiting China must make health declaration with the health quarantine departments of the customs and well cooperate in such health quarantine work as body temperature monitoring, medical check, and medical screening.

2. 《中华人民共和国国境卫生检疫法》

第十六条　国境卫生检疫机关有权要求入境、出境的人员填写健康申明卡，出示某种传染病的预防接种证书、健康证明或者其他有关证件。

2. Frontier Health and Quarantine Law of the People's Republic of China

Article 16　Frontier health and quarantine offices shall be authorized to require persons on entry or exit to complete a health declaration form and produce certificates of vaccination against certain infectious diseases, a health certificate or other relevant documents.

3. 《中华人民共和国国境卫生检疫法实施细则》

第一百条　受入境、出境检疫的人员，必须根据检疫医师的要求，如实填报健康申明卡，出示某种有效的传染病预防接种证书、健康证明或者其他有关证件。

3. Detailed Rules for the Implementation of the Frontier Health and Quarantine Law of the People's Republic of China

Article 100　The people subject to entry or exit quarantine inspection are required to fill out health card as required by the quarantine physician, to present a valid certificate of inoculation against epidemic diseases, bill of health or other related certificate.

4.1.2 不如实填报健康申明卡等行为的法律责任
Legal liability for acts such as untruthful declaration

1.《中华人民共和国国境卫生检疫法》

第二十条 对违反本法规定，有下列行为之一的单位或者个人，国境卫生检疫机关可以根据情节轻重，给予警告或者罚款：

（一）逃避检疫，向国境卫生检疫机关隐瞒真实情况的；

（二）入境的人员未经国境卫生检疫机关许可，擅自上下交通工具，或者装卸行李、货物、邮包等物品，不听劝阻的。

罚款全部上缴国库。

第二十一条 当事人对国境卫生检疫机关给予的罚款决定不服的，可以在接到通知之日起十五日内，向当地人民法

1. Frontier Health and Quarantine Law of the People's Republic of China

Article 20 A frontier health and quarantine office may warn or fine, according to the circumstances, any unit or individual that has violated the provisions of this Law by committing any of the following acts:

（1）evading quarantine inspection or withholding the truth in reports to the frontier health and quarantine office;

（2）embarking on or disembarking from conveyances upon entry, or loading or unloading articles such as baggage, goods or postal parcels, without the permission of a frontier health and quarantine office and refusing to listen to the office's advice against such acts.

All fines thus collected shall be turned over to the state treasury.

Article 21 If a concerned party refuses to obey a decision on a fine made by a frontier health and quarantine office, he may, within 15 days after receiving notice

院起诉。逾期不起诉又不履行的，国境卫生检疫机关可以申请人民法院强制执行。

第二十二条　违反本法规定，引起检疫传染病传播或者有引起检疫传染病传播严重危险的，依照刑法有关规定追究刑事责任。

2.《中华人民共和国国境卫生检疫法实施细则》

第一百零九条、一百一十条规定，拒绝接受检疫或者抵制卫生监督，拒不接受卫生处理①的；应当受行政处罚，处以警告或者 100 元以上 5000 元以下的罚款。

第一百零九条、第一百一十条规定，隐瞒疫情或者伪造情节的应当受行政处罚，处以 1000 元以上 1 万元以下的罚

of the fine, file a lawsuit in a local people's court. The frontier health and quarantine office may apply to the people's court for mandatory enforcement of a decision if the concerned party neither files a lawsuit nor obeys the decision within the 15-day term.

Article 22　If a quarantinable infectious disease is caused to spread or is in great danger of being spread as a result of a violation of the provisions of this Law, criminal responsibility shall be investigated according to the relevant provisions of the Criminal Law.

2. Detailed Rules for the Implementation of the Frontier Health and Quarantine Law of the People's Republic of China

Article 109 and Article 110 specify that those who refuse to undergo quarantine inspection or sanitary supervision, or refuse to allow sanitation measures to be taken shall get a warning or a fine ranging from RMB 100 yuan to RMB 5,000 yuan.

Article 109 and Article 110 specify that those who hide the truth of quarantine epidemic disease from the health and quarantine organ or falsify the details of the

---

① "卫生处理"指隔离、留验和就地诊验等医学措施，以及消毒、除鼠、除虫等卫生措施。

款。

3.《中华人民共和国刑法》

第三百三十二条 【妨害国境卫生检疫罪】违反国境卫生检疫规定，引起检疫传染病传播或者有传播严重危险的，处三年以下有期徒刑或者拘役，并处或者单处罚金。

4.《关于进一步加强国境卫生检疫工作 依法惩治妨害国境卫生检疫违法犯罪的意见》的通知

根据最高人民法院、最高人民检察院、公安部、司法部、海关总署于 2022 年 3 月 16 日联合发布的《关于进一步加强国境卫生检疫工作 依法惩治妨害国境卫生检疫违法犯罪的意见》，实施以下六类妨害国境卫生检疫行为，如果引起鼠疫、霍乱、黄热病以及新冠肺炎等国务院确定和公布的其他检疫传染病传播或者有传播严重危

situation will get a fine ranging from RMB 10,000 yuan to RMB 10,000 yuan.

3. Criminal Law of the People's Republic of China

Article 332 [crime of obstructing frontier health and quarantine] Whoever, in violation of the provisions on frontier health and quarantine, causes the spread or a grave danger of the spread of a quarantinable infectious disease shall be sentenced to fixed-term imprisonment of not more than three years or criminal detention and shall also, or shall only, be fined.

4. Opinions on Further Strengthening Frontier Health and Quarantine Efforts as well as Lawfully Punishing Illegal and Criminal Activities that Impair Frontier Health and Quarantine Regulation

According to Notice by the Supreme People's Court, the Supreme People's Procuratorate, the Ministry of Public Security, and the General Administration of Customs of the Opinions on Further Strengthening Frontier Health and Quarantine Efforts as well as Lawfully Punishing Illegal and Criminal Activities that Impair Frontier Health and Quarantine Regulation on March 16, 2022, the following 6 types of activities that may cause

险的，将依照《中华人民共和国刑法》第三百三十二条规定，以妨害国境卫生检疫罪定罪处罚：

1. 检疫传染病染疫人①或者染疫嫌疑人②拒绝执行海关依照国境卫生检疫法等法律法规提出的健康申报、体温监测、医学巡查、流行病学调查、医学排查、采样等卫生检疫措施，或者隔离③、留验④、就地诊验⑤、转诊等卫生处理措施的；

or risk causing the spread of plague, cholera, yellow fever, COVID-19 or other quarantinable communicable diseases identified by the State Council, will constitute the crime of impairing border health quarantine, and the perpetrator will be convicted and punished in accordance with Article 332 of the Criminal Law of the People's Pepublic of China.

1. A person infected or suspected to be infected with a quarantinable communicable disease refuses to comply with health and quarantine measures, such as health declaration, body temperature monitoring, health assessment, epidemiological investigation, medical screening, sampling, or isolation, medical observation, on-site examination or referral, which are required by the Customs according to the Frontier Health and Quarantine Law of the People's Republic of China and other laws and regulations.

---

① "染疫人"指正在患检疫传染病的人，或者经卫生检疫机关初步诊断，认为已经感染检疫传染病或者已经处于检疫传染病潜伏期的人。

② "染疫嫌疑人"指接触过检疫传染病的感染环境，并且可能传播检疫传染病的人。

③ "隔离"指将染疫人收留在指定的处所，限制其活动并进行治疗，直到消除传染病传播的危险。

④ "留验"指将染疫嫌疑人收留在指定的处所进行诊察和检验。

⑤ "就地诊验"指一个人在卫生检疫机关指定的期间，到就近的卫生检疫机关或者其他医疗卫生单位去接受诊察和检验；或者卫生检疫机关、其他医疗卫生单位到该人员的居留地，对其进行诊察和检验。

2. 检疫传染病染疫人或者染疫嫌疑人采取不如实填报健康申明卡等方式隐瞒疫情，或者伪造、涂改检疫单、证等方式伪造情节的；

3. 知道或者应当知道实施审批管理的微生物、人体组织、生物制品、血液及其制品等特殊物品可能造成检疫传染病传播，未经审批仍逃避检疫，携运、寄递出入境的；

4. 出入境交通工具上发现有检疫传染病染疫人或者染疫嫌疑人，交通工具负责人拒绝接受卫生检疫或者拒不接受卫生处理的；

5. 来自检疫传染病流行国家、地区的出入境交通工具上出现非意外伤害死亡且死因不明的人员，交通工具负责人故意隐瞒情况的；

6. 其他拒绝执行海关依照国境卫生检疫法等法律法规提

2. A person infected or suspected to be infected with a quarantinable communicable disease conceals the fact of infection by untruthfully filling out the Exit/Entry Health Declaration Form or falsifying quarantine documentation.

3. A person, who is or should be aware that microorganisms, human tissues, biological products, blood, blood products and other special articles subject to approval management may cause the spread of quarantinable communicable diseases, evades quarantine and carries/mails such articles across the border without approval.

4. A person infected or suspected to be infected with a quarantinable communicable disease is found aboard an entry/exit conveyance, and the supervisor of the conveyance refuses to follow the health and quarantine protocol.

5. When there is non-accidental death for unknown reasons on a conveyance travelling from countries or regions with quarantinable communicable diseases, and the supervisor of the conveyance conceals the truth.

6. Refusal in any other form to comply with customs health and quarantine

出的检疫措施的。

measures that are taken in line with the Frontier Health and Quarantine Law of the People's Republic of China and other laws and regulations.

4.2　疫情防控涉及的法规制度
Laws and regulations concerning epidemic prevention and control

4.2.1　中华人民共和国宪法
Constitution of the People's Republic of China

第三十二条　中华人民共和国保护在中国境内的外国人的合法权利和利益，在中国境内的外国人必须遵守中华人民共和国的法律。

Article 32　The People's Republic of China protects the lawful rights and interests of foreigners within Chinese territory; foreigners on Chinese territory must abide by the laws of the People's Republic of China.

4.2.2　中华人民共和国国境卫生检疫法
Frontier Health and Quarantine Law of the People's Republic of China

第十二条　国境卫生检疫机关对检疫传染病染疫人必须立即将其隔离，隔离期限根据医学检查结果确定；对检疫传染病染疫嫌疑人应当将其留验，留验期限根据该传染病的潜伏

Article 12　A person having a quarantinable infectious disease shall be placed in isolation by the frontier health and quarantine office for a period determined by the results of the medical examination, while a person suspected of having a

期确定。

quarantinable infectious disease shall be kept for inspection for a period determined by the incubation period of such disease.

4.2.3 中华人民共和国传染病防治法
Law of the People's Republic of China on Prevention and Treatment of Infectious Diseases

第三十九条 医疗机构发现甲类传染病时，应当及时采取下列措施：

（一）对病人、病原携带者，予以隔离治疗，隔离期限根据医学检查结果确定；

（二）对疑似病人，确诊前在指定场所单独隔离治疗；

（三）对医疗机构内的病人、病原携带者、疑似病人的密切接触者，在指定场所进行医学观察和采取其他必要的预防措施。

拒绝隔离治疗或者隔离期未满擅自脱离隔离治疗的，可以由公安机关协助医疗机构采

Article 39　When finding an infectious disease under Class A, the medical agency shall immediately take the following measures:

（1）to isolate the patients and pathogen carriers for treatment, and to determine the period of isolation according to the results of medical examination;

（2）to treat suspected patients individually in isolation at designated places until a definite diagnosis is made; and

（3）to keep the persons in close contact with the patients, pathogen carriers or suspected patients in medical agencies under medical observation at designated places and to take other necessary preventive measures.

With regard to the persons who refuse treatment in isolation or, before the expiration of the period of isolation, break

取强制隔离治疗措施。

医疗机构发现乙类或者丙类传染病病人，应当根据病情采取必要的治疗和控制传播措施。

医疗机构对本单位内被传染病病原体污染的场所、物品以及医疗废物，必须依照法律、法规的规定实施消毒和无害化处置。

第四十条 疾病预防控制机构发现传染病疫情或者接到传染病疫情报告时，应当及时采取下列措施：

（一）对传染病疫情进行流行病学调查，根据调查情况提出划定疫点、疫区的建议，对被污染的场所进行卫生处理，对密切接触者，在指定场所进行医学观察和采取其他必要的预防措施，并向卫生行政部门

away from treatment in isolation without approval, the public security organs may assist the medical agencies by taking compulsory measures for treatment in isolation.

When medical agencies find patients of infectious diseases under Class B or C, they shall take necessary measures for treatment and for control of their spread according to the patients' conditions.

With regard to the places and objects contaminated by pathogens of infectious diseases as well as the medical wastes within their own units, medical agencies shall, in accordance with the provisions of laws and regulations, carry out disinfection and innocent treatment.

Article 40 When finding epidemic situation of infectious diseases or receiving reports on such situation, the disease prevention and control institutions shall immediately take the following measures：

（1） to make epidemiological investigation on the epidemic situation of infectious diseases and, on the basis of the findings after such investigation, to put forth proposals for the delimitation of epidemic spots and areas; to give sanitary treatment to the contaminated places, to keep the

提出疫情控制方案；

（二）传染病暴发、流行时，对疫点、疫区进行卫生处理，向卫生行政部门提出疫情控制方案，并按照卫生行政部门的要求采取措施；

（三）指导下级疾病预防控制机构实施传染病预防、控制措施，组织、指导有关单位对传染病疫情的处理。

第四十一条 对已经发生甲类传染病病例的场所或者该场所内的特定区域的人员，所在地的县级以上地方人民政府可以实施隔离措施，并同时向上一级人民政府报告；接到报告的上级人民政府应当即时作出是否批准的决定。上级人民

persons in close contact under medical observation at the designated places and to take other necessary preventive measures, and to put forth schemes for control of the epidemic situation to health administration departments;

（2）when an infectious disease breaks out and prevails, to give sanitary treatment to epidemic spots and areas, to put forth schemes for control of the epidemic situation to the health administration departments, and to take measures in accordance with the requirements of health administration departments; and

（3）to direct the disease prevention and control institutions at lower levels in implementing the measures for prevention and control of infectious diseases and to coordinate efforts and direct relevant units in handling the epidemic situation of infectious diseases.

Article 41　With respect to the places where there are cases of infectious diseases under Class A or to the persons in the special areas within such places, the local people's governments at or above the county level where the above places are located may carry out isolation measures and, at the same time, report the matter to the people's

政府作出不予批准决定的，实施隔离措施的人民政府应当立即解除隔离措施。

在隔离期间，实施隔离措施的人民政府应当对被隔离人员提供生活保障；被隔离人员有工作单位的，所在单位不得停止支付其隔离期间的工作报酬。

隔离措施的解除，由原决定机关决定并宣布。

governments at the next higher level; and upon receiving such report, the people's governments at the higher level shall immediately make a decision on whether to approve the measures or not. Where the people's governments at the higher level decide not to approve the measures, the people's governments that have taken isolation measures shall immediately withdraw such measures.

During the period of isolation, the people's governments that take isolation measures shall guarantee the daily necessities of the persons under isolation; and if such persons have their own units, the units, which they belong to, shall not stop the payment of their wages during the period of isolation.

Withdrawal of isolation measures shall be subject to decision and announcement by the organ that originally makes the decision to take the measures.

4.2.4 中华人民共和国出境入境管理法
Exit and Entry Administration Law of the People's Republic of China

第三条 ……在中国境内

Article 3 …The legitimate rights and

的外国人的合法权益受法律保护。在中国境内的外国人应当遵守中国法律，不得危害中国国家安全、损害社会公共利益、破坏社会公共秩序。

第二十一条　外国人有下列情形之一的，不予签发签证：

……

（二）患有严重精神障碍、传染性肺结核病或者有可能对公共卫生造成重大危害的其他传染病的；

……

第六十一条　外国人有下列情形之一的，不适用拘留审查，可以限制其活动范围：

（一）患有严重疾病的；

……

interests of foreigners in China shall be protected by laws. Foreigners in China shall abide by the Chinese laws, and shall not endanger China's national security, harm public interests and disrupt social and public order.

Article 21　Under any of the following circumstances, visas shall not be issued to foreigners:

…

（2）Is suffering from serious mental disorders, infectious tuberculosis or other infectious diseases that may severely jeopardize the public health;

…

Article 61　Under any of the following circumstances, detention for investigation is not applicable to foreigners, however their movements may be restricted:

（1）Suffer from serious diseases;

…

4.2.5　中华人民共和国治安管理处罚法
Law of the People's Republic of China on Penalties for Administration of Public Security

第二十五条　有下列行为之一的，处五日以上十日以下

Article 25　A person who commits any of the following acts shall be detained for

拘留，可以并处五百元以下罚款；情节较轻的，处五日以下拘留或者五百元以下罚款：

（一）散布谣言，谎报险情、疫情、警情或者以其他方法故意扰乱公共秩序的；

……

第五十条　有下列行为之一的，处警告或者二百元以下罚款；情节严重的，处五日以上十日以下拘留，可以并处五百元以下罚款：

（一）拒不执行人民政府在紧急状态情况下依法发布的决定、命令的；

（二）阻碍国家机关工作人员依法执行职务的；

……

not less than 5 days but not more than 10 days and may, in addition, be fined not more than 500 yuan; if the circumstances are relatively minor, he shall be detained for not more than 5 days or be fined not more than 500 yuan:

（1） intentionally disturbing public order by spreading rumors, making false reports of dangerous situations or epidemic situations, raising false alarms or by other means;

…

Article 50　A person who commits any of the following acts shall be given a warning or be fined not more than 200 yuan; if the circumstances are serious, he shall be detained for not less than 5 days but not more than 10 days, and may, in addition, be fined not more than 500 yuan:

（1） refusing to carry out the decision or order issued according to law by the people's government in the state of emergency;

（2） obstructing the working personnel of state organs from performing their duties according to law;

…

4.2.6　中华人民共和国刑法
Criminal Law of the People's Republic of China

第一百一十四条　【放火罪、决水罪、爆炸罪、投放危险物质罪、以危险方法危害公共安全罪（之一）】放火、决水、爆炸以及投放毒害性、放射性、传染病病原体等物质或者以其他危险方法危害公共安全，尚未造成严重后果的，处三年以上十年以下有期徒刑。

第一百一十五条　【放火罪、决水罪、爆炸罪、投放危险物质罪、以危险方法危害公共安全罪（之二）】放火、决水、爆炸以及投放毒害性、放射性、传染病病原体等物质或者以其他危险方法致人重伤、死亡或者使公私财产遭受重大损失的，处十年以上有期徒刑、无期徒刑或者死刑。

Article 114　[arson, crime of breaching a dike, crime of causing explosion, crime of spreading poison and crimes against public security by other dangerous means] Whoever commits arson, breaches dikes, causes explosions, spreads pathogen of infectious diseases, poisonous or radioactive substances or other substances, or uses other dangerous means to endanger public security, but hasn't caused any serious consequences, shall be sentenced to fixed-term imprisonment of no less than three years but no more than ten years.

Article 115　[arson, crime of breaching a dike, crime of causing explosion, crime of spreading poison and crimes against public security by other dangerous means] Whoever commits arson, breaches dikes, causes explosions, spreads pathogens of infectious diseases, poisonous or radioactive substances or other substances, or uses other dangerous means to have inflicted any serious injury or death on people or caused heavy losses of public or private property, shall be sentenced to fixed-term

过失犯前款罪的，处三年以上七年以下有期徒刑；情节较轻的，处三年以下有期徒刑或者拘役。

第二百七十七条 【妨害公务罪】以暴力、威胁方法阻碍国家机关工作人员依法执行职务的，处三年以下有期徒刑、拘役、管制或者罚金。

……

在自然灾害和突发事件中，以暴力、威胁方法阻碍红十字会工作人员依法履行职责的，依照第一款的规定处罚。

第三百三十条 【妨害传染病防治罪】违反传染病防治法的规定，有下列情形之一，

imprisonment of no less than ten years, life imprisonment or death.

Whoever negligently commits the crimes in the preceding paragraph shall be sentenced to fixed-term imprisonment of not less than three years but not more than seven years; if the circumstances are minor, he shall be sentenced to fixed-term imprisonment of not more than three years, or criminal detention.

Article 277 [crime of disrupting public service] Whoever by means of violence or threat, obstructs a functionary of a state organ from carrying out his functions according to law shall be sentenced to fixed-term imprisonment of not more than three years, criminal detention, or public surveillance or be fined.

...

Whoever during natural calamities or emergencies obstructs, by means of violence or threat, the workers of the Red Cross Society from performing their functions and duties according to law shall be punished in accordance with the provisions of the first paragraph.

Article 330 [crime of impairing infectious disease prevention] Whoever, in violation of the provisions of the Law on

引起甲类传染病传播或者有传播严重危险的，处三年以下有期徒刑或者拘役；后果特别严重的，处三年以上七年以下有期徒刑：

……

（四）拒绝执行卫生防疫机构依照传染病防治法提出的预防、控制措施的。

第三百三十二条 【妨害国境卫生检疫罪】违反国境卫生检疫规定，引起检疫传染病传播或者有传播严重危险的，处三年以下有期徒刑或者拘役，并处或者单处罚金。

Prevention and Treatment of Infectious Diseases, commits any of the following acts and thus causes the spread or a grave danger of the spread of an A Class infectious disease shall be sentenced to fixed-term imprisonment of not more than three years or criminal detention; if the consequences are especially serious, he shall be sentenced to fixed-term imprisonment of not less than three years but not more than seven years.

…

（4）refusal to execute the preventive and control measures proposed by the health and anti-epidemic agencies according to the Law on Prevention and Treatment of Infectious Diseases.

Article 332 [crime of obstructing frontier health and quarantine] Whoever, in violation of the provisions on frontier health and quarantine, causes the spread or a grave danger of the spread of a quarantinable infectious disease shall be sentenced to fixed-term imprisonment of not more than three years or criminal detention and shall also, or shall only, be fined.

4.2.7 突发公共卫生事件应急条例
Regulations on Emergency Response to Unexpected Public Health Incidents

第四十四条　在突发事件中需要接受隔离治疗、医学观察措施的病人、疑似病人和传染病病人密切接触者在卫生行政主管部门或者有关机构采取医学措施时应当予以配合；拒绝配合的，由公安机关依法协助强制执行。

Article 44　In the emergent hazard, patients, suspected patients or persons in close contact with patients of infectious diseases, who are required to be isolated for medical treatment, or be subject to medical observation, shall be cooperative when the competent health administrative departments or relevant institutions take sanitary measures. If they refuse to do so, the public security organs shall assist in enforcing these measures according to law.

Words & Expressions

quarantine/ˈkwɔːrəntiːn/ n. 隔离

procuratorate/ˈprɒkjʊəreɪtərɪt/ n. 代理人之职，检察院

calamity/kəˈlæməti/ n. 灾祸，不幸之事

tuberculosis/tuːˌbɜːrkjəˈloʊsɪs/ n. 肺结核，[医]结核病，痨，痨病

jeopardize/ˈdʒepərdaɪz/ v. 危及，损害，使陷入险境或受伤，使……遇险

inflict/ɪnˈflɪkt/ v. 把……强加给，使承受，遭受，给予（打击等），处以刑罚，加刑

negligent/ˈneglɪdʒənt/ adj. 疏忽的，粗心大意的，不留心的，懒散的

5

口岸疫情防控文摘

Sentences and Articles on
Fighting the Epidemic at Ports

※※※※※※※※※※※※※※※※※※※※※※※※※※※※※※※※※※※※

导读：新冠肺炎疫情在全球暴发以来，已构成国际关注的突发公共卫生事件。面对冲击，世界各国（地区）开展了抗击新冠肺炎疫情这场"没有硝烟的战役"。在"抗疫"过程中，中国始终把人民群众生命安全和身体健康放在首位，并将其作为应对疫情的第一原则。在各级政府统筹协调有力、医疗资源调配合理、全民积极配合的基础上，国内疫情得到了有效控制。

中国在世界范围内率先采取有效的防控措施，确保了人民的生命安全，为全球取得"抗疫"胜利提供了宝贵的中国经验，同时展现出的以人为本的"抗疫"精神更值得在世界各国推广。

中国还率先向有需要的发展中国家提供疫苗，截至 2022 年 3 月，中国对外提供疫苗量超过 21 亿剂，成为世界上对外提供疫苗量最多的国家。此外，中国还向有需要的国家（地区）和国际组织提供检测试剂等各种医疗卫生产品，在不同维度为世界抗击新冠肺炎疫情做出了巨大贡献。

当前，新冠肺炎疫情仍在全球起伏反复，世界各国（地区）同处一个"地球村"，安危与共、休戚相关，需携手应对。中国政府一直提倡国际社会同心协力，通过加强国际合作应对全球公共卫生安全危机，建立全球公共卫生及传染病防控合作机制。

本章内容为疫情防控文摘，主要摘录了国内外有关疫情防控的官方文件、新闻、评论或文章片段，方便读者学习。

※※※※※※※※※※※※※※※※※※※※※※※※※※※※※※※※※※※※

5.1 国内疫情防控 China's fight against the epidemic①

1. 新冠肺炎是近百年来人类遭遇的影响范围最广的全球性大流行病，对全世界是一次严重危机和严峻考验。人类生命安全和健康面临重大威胁。

2. 这是一场全人类与病毒的"战争"。面对前所未知、突如其来、来势汹汹的疫情，中国果断打响疫情防控阻击战，把人民生命安全和身体健康放在第一位，以坚定果敢的勇气和决心，采取最全面、最严格、最彻底的防控措施，有效阻断病毒传播链条。14 亿中国人民坚韧奉献、团结协作，构筑起同心战"疫"的坚固防线，彰显了人民的伟大力量。

3. 中国始终秉持人类命运共同体理念，肩负大国担当，同其他国家并肩作战、共克时

1. The COVID-19 is the most extensive global pandemic to afflict humanity in a century, a serious crisis for the entire world, and a daunting challenge. It poses a grave threat to human life and health.

2. This is a war that humanity has to fight and win. Facing this unknown, unexpected, and devastating disease, China launched a resolute battle to prevent and control its spread. Making people's lives and health its first priority, China adopted extensive, stringent, and thorough containment measures, and has for now succeeded in cutting all channels for the transmission of the virus. 1.4 billion Chinese people have exhibited enormous tenacity and solidarity in erecting a defensive rampart that demonstrates their power in the face of such natural disasters.

3. Having forged the idea that the world is a global community of shared future, and believing that it must act as a

---

① 第 5.1 节内容均摘自国务院新闻办公室 2020 年 6 月发布的《抗击新冠肺炎疫情的中国行动》白皮书（中英文版）。

艰。中国本着依法、公开、透明、负责任的态度，第一时间向国际社会通报疫情信息，毫无保留地同各方分享防控和救治经验。中国对疫情给各国人民带来的苦难感同身受，尽己所能向国际社会提供人道主义援助，支持全球抗击疫情。

4. 新冠肺炎疫情是中华人民共和国成立以来发生的传播速度最快、感染范围最广、防控难度最大的一次重大突发公共卫生事件，对中国是一次危机，也是一次大考。

5. 在中国共产党的领导下，全国上下贯彻"坚定信心、同舟共济、科学防治、精准施策"的总要求，打响抗击疫情的人民战争、总体战、阻击战。

6. 经过艰苦卓绝的努力，

responsible member, China has fought shoulder to shoulder with the rest of the world. In an open, transparent, and responsible manner and in accordance with the law, China gave timely notification to the international community of the onset of a new coronavirus, and shared without reserve its experience in containing the spread of the virus and treating the infected. China has great empathy with victims all over the world, and has done all it can to provide humanitarian aid in support of the international community's endeavors to stem the pandemic.

4. The COVID-19 epidemic is a major public health emergency. The virus has spread faster and wider than any other since the founding of the People's Republic of China in 1949, and has proven to be the most difficult to contain. It is both a crisis and a major test for China.

5. Under the leadership of the CPC, the whole nation has followed the general principle of "remaining confident, coming together in solidarity, adopting a science-based approach, and taking targeted measures", and waged an all-out people's war on the virus.

6. Through painstaking efforts and

中国付出巨大代价和牺牲，有力扭转了疫情局势，用一个多月的时间初步遏制了疫情蔓延势头，用两个月左右的时间将本土每日新增病例控制在个位数以内，用三个月左右的时间取得了"武汉保卫战""湖北保卫战"的决定性成果，疫情防控阻击战取得重大战略成果，维护了人民生命安全和身体健康，为维护地区和世界公共卫生安全做出了重要贡献。

7. 中国疾控中心、中国医学科学院作为国家卫生健康委的指定机构，向世界卫生组织提交新型冠状病毒基因组序列信息，在全球流感共享数据库（GISAID）发布，全球共享。

8. 2020 年 1 月 20 日，国务院总理李克强主持召开国务院常务会议，进一步部署疫情防控工作，并根据《中华人民共和国传染病防治法》将新冠肺炎纳入乙类传染病，采取甲类传染病管理措施。

tremendous sacrifice, and having paid a heavy price, China has succeeded in turning the situation around. In little more than a single month, the rising spread of the virus was contained; in around two months, the daily increase in domestic coronavirus cases had fallen to single digits; and in approximately three months, a decisive victory was secured in the battle to defend Hubei Province and its capital city of Wuhan. With these strategic achievements, China has protected its people's lives, safety and health, and made a significant contribution to safeguarding regional and global public health.

7. China CDC, the CAMS, as designated agencies of the NHC, submitted to the WHO the genome sequence of the novel coronavirus(2019-nCoV）, which was published by the Global Initiative on Sharing All Influenza Data to be shared globally.

8. On January 20, 2020, during an executive meeting of the State Council, Premier Li Keqiang decided to take more steps for epidemic prevention and control. A decision was taken to classify the novel coronavirus pneumonia as a Class B infectious disease in compliance with the

Law of the People's Republic of China on Prevention and Treatment of Infectious Diseases, but to apply to it the preventive and control measures for a Class A infectious disease.

9. 中共中央总书记习近平主持召开中共中央政治局常务委员会会议，明确提出"坚定信心、同舟共济、科学防治、精准施策"总要求，强调坚决打赢疫情防控阻击战；指出湖北省要把疫情防控工作作为当前头等大事，采取更严格的措施，内防扩散、外防输出；强调要按照集中患者、集中专家、集中资源、集中救治"四集中"原则，将重症病例集中到综合力量强的定点医疗机构进行救治，及时收治所有确诊病人。

9. Xi Jinping chaired a meeting of the Standing Committee of the Political Bureau of the CPC Central Committee. He called for resolute efforts to win the battle to contain the virus with "confidence and solidarity, a science-based approach and targeted measures". He urged Hubei to make epidemic control its top priority and apply more rigorous measures to stem the spread of the virus within the province and beyond. All confirmed patients, he said, must be hospitalized without delay, and severe cases must be sent to designated hospitals with sufficient medical resources so that they could be treated by medical experts.

10. 中国政府指出，要坚持底线思维，做好较长时间应对外部环境变化的思想准备和工作准备；强调"外防输入、内防反弹"，防控工作决不能放松；强调要抓好无症状感染者精准防控，把疫情防控网扎得更密更牢，堵住所有可能导

10. Chinese government reiterated the need to stay alert against potential risks and be prepared, both in thinking and action, to respond to long-term changes in the external environment. He warned against any relaxation of the efforts to both stop inbound cases and forestall domestic resurgence of cases. Targeted measures

致疫情反弹的漏洞；强调要加强陆海口岸疫情防控，最大限度减少境外输入关联本地病例。

11. 2020 年 4 月 29 日以来，境内疫情总体呈零星散发状态，局部地区出现散发病例引起的聚集性疫情，境外输入病例基本得到控制，疫情积极向好态势持续巩固，全国疫情防控进入常态化。

12. 实施分级、分类、动态精准防控。全国推行分区分级精准施策防控策略，以县域为单位，依据人口、发病情况综合研判，划分低、中、高疫情风险等级，分区分级实施差异化防控，并根据疫情形势及时动态调整名单，采取对应防控措施。

should be taken to manage asymptomatic cases, build a strong line of defense and plug any loopholes that might cause a resurgence of the virus. Control at land and sea points of entry should be tightened to minimize domestic cases caused by inbound arrivals carrying the virus.

11. Since April 29, 2020, sporadic cases have been reported on the mainland, resulting in case clusters in some locations. Inbound cases are generally under control. The positive momentum in COVID-19 control has thus been locked in, and nationwide virus control is now being conducted on an ongoing basis.

12. A multi-level, category-specific, dynamic and targeted approach was adopted. China also applied a region-specific, multi-level approach to epidemic prevention and control. To better prevent and control the epidemic, each region at or above the county level was classified by risk level on the basis of a comprehensive evaluation of factors such as population and number of infections in a given period of time. There are three levels of risk: low, medium, and high. Regions could take measures according to the risk level, which was dynamic and adjusted in light of the

evolving situation.

13. 低风险区严防输入，全面恢复生产生活秩序；中风险区外防输入、内防扩散，尽快全面恢复生产生活秩序；高风险区内防扩散、外防输出、严格管控，集中精力抓疫情防控。

13. In response to COVID-19, a low-risk region was requested to remain vigilant against any potential inbound transmission while fully restoring normal order in work and daily life; a medium-risk region had to prevent inbound and local transmission while restoring normal work and daily life as soon as possible; and a region classified as high-risk was obliged to prevent any spread in its jurisdiction or beyond, enforce strict control measures, and focus on containment.

14. 本土疫情形势稳定后，以省域为单元在疫情防控常态化条件下加快恢复生产生活秩序，健全及时发现、快速处置、精准管控、有效救治的常态化防控机制。

14. Once the situation stabilized, provincial-level authorities could step up efforts to restore order in work and daily life in areas under their jurisdiction, while adapting to the new normal of COVID-19 control by establishing a sound long-term epidemic response system that ensures early detection, quick response, targeted prevention and control, and effective treatment.

15. 做好重点场所、重点单位、重点人群聚集性疫情防控和处置，加强老年人、儿童、孕产妇、学生、医务人员等重点人群健康管理，加强医疗机构、社区、办公场所、商场超市、客运场站、交通运输工具、托幼机构、中小学校、大专院

15. Appropriate measures were implemented to prevent any cluster outbreaks in key locations, major organizations, and priority population groups, and manage the aftermath of any such outbreaks. The elderly, children, pregnant women, students, and health workers were to be well protected as a

校以及养老机构、福利院、精神卫生医疗机构、救助站等特殊场所的管控，覆盖全人群、全场所、全社区，不留死角、不留空白、不留隐患。

priority. Health management of priority population groups was enhanced. Protective measures were intensified in medical facilities, communities, office buildings, shopping malls and supermarkets, passenger terminals, transport vehicles, child-care centers and kindergartens, elementary and secondary schools, colleges and universities, nursing homes, charity houses, mental health institutions, and first-aid stations. These measures were implemented nationwide, covering all population groups, locations, and communities, and leaving no areas unattended and no hidden dangers unaddressed.

16. 针对输入性疫情，严格落实国境卫生检疫措施，强化从"国门"到"家门"的全链条、闭环式管理，持续抓紧抓实抓细外防输入、内防反弹工作。

16. To control any inbound infections from overseas, China has strictly enforced its border health and quarantine rules to ensure a full, closed cycle of management of all arrivals, from their entry at the border to the doorstep of where they would stay. Sustained, meticulous efforts have been made to prevent both inbound cases and a recurrence in domestic cases.

17. 社区工作者、基层干部、下沉干部、公安民警、海关关员不辞辛苦、日夜值守，为保护人民生命安全牺牲奉献。

17. Community workers, primary and community-level officials, officials sent to work in communities, police, and customs officers worked day and night to protect

400 万名社区工作者奋战在全国 65 万个城乡社区中，监测疫情、测量体温、排查人员、宣传政策、防疫消杀，认真细致，尽职尽责，守好疫情防控"第一关口"。公安民警及辅警驻守医院、转运病人、巡逻街道、维护秩序，面对急难险重任务勇挑重担，130 多人牺牲在工作岗位。海关关员依法履行卫生检疫职责，筑牢口岸检疫防线。

18. 中国及时向国际社会通报疫情信息，交流防控经验，为全球防疫提供了基础性支持。

19. 中国与多个国际和区域组织开展 70 多次疫情防控交流活动。国家卫生健康委汇编诊疗和防控方案并翻译成 3 个语种，分享给全球 180 多个国家、10 多个国际和区域组织参

lives and public safety. Some 4 million community workers are working in around 650, 000 urban and rural communities, monitoring the situation, taking body temperatures, screening for infection, disseminating government policies, and sanitizing neighborhoods. Dedicated and responsible, they have meticulously protected their communities from the virus. Police and auxiliary police officers handled emergent, difficult, dangerous, and burdensome tasks such as guarding hospitals, transporting patients, and patrolling the streets to maintain order. More than 130 have died in the line of duty. Customs officers have applied the law and carried out quarantine and other health-related duties, preventing the virus from entering the country.

18. China has provided support for global virus prevention and control by promptly sharing information and experience with the international community.

19. China has conducted more than 70 exchanges with international and regional organizations. The National Health Commission (NHC) has worked out diagnosis, treatment, prevention and control solutions, had them translated into three

照使用，并与世界卫生组织联合举办"分享新冠肺炎防治中国经验国际通报会"。

20. 2020年3月1日至5月31日，中国向200个国家和地区出口防疫物资，其中，口罩706亿只，防护服3.4亿套，护目镜1.15亿个，呼吸机9.67万台，检测试剂盒2.25亿人份，红外线测温仪4029万台，出口规模呈明显增长态势，有力支持了相关国家疫情防控。

21. 当前，疫情在全球持续蔓延。中国为被病毒夺去生命和在抗击疫情中牺牲的人们深感痛惜，向争分夺秒抢救生命、遏制疫情的人们深表敬意，向不幸感染病毒、正在进行治疗的人们表达祝愿。中国坚信，国际社会同舟共济、守望相助，就一定能够战胜疫情，走出人类历史上这段艰难时刻，迎来人类更加美好的明天。

languages, and shared them with over 180 countries and more than 10 international and regional organizations. Together with the WHO, China held a "Briefing on China's Experience on COVID-19 Response".

20. From March 1 to May 31, 2020, China exported protective materials to 200 countries and regions, among which there were more than 70.6 billion masks, 340 million protective suits, 115 million pairs of goggles, 96,700 ventilators, 225 million test kits, and 40.29 million infrared thermometers. China's growing exports provide strong support for the prevention and control efforts of affected countries.

21. The virus is currently wreaking havoc throughout the world. China grieves for those who have been killed and those who have sacrificed their lives in the fight, extends the greatest respect to those who are struggling to save lives, and offers true moral support to those who are infected and receiving treatment. China firmly believes that as long as all countries unite and cooperate to mount a collective response, the international community will succeed in overcoming the pandemic, and will emerge from this dark moment in human history into a brighter future.

Words & Expressions

afflict/əˈflɪkt/ v. 折磨，使痛苦

daunting/ˈdɔːntɪŋ/ adj. 令人畏惧的，使人气馁的，令人却步的

resolute/ˈrezəluːt/ adj. 坚决的，刚毅的，不动摇的

tenacity/təˈnæsəti/ n. [物] 韧性，韧度，固执，坚持，不屈不挠，黏性

rampart/ˈræmpɑːrt/ n. （城堡等周围宽阔的）防御土墙，防御，保护

wreak/riːk/ v. 造成（巨大的破坏或伤害），施行（报复）

havoc/ˈhævək/ n. 灾难，混乱；v. 严重破坏

arduous/ˈɑːrdʒuəs/ adj. 努力的，艰巨的，难克服的，陡峭的

indomitable/ɪnˈdɑːmɪtəbl/ adj. 不屈不挠的，不服输的，不气馁的

bastion/ˈbæstʃən/ n. 堡垒，棱堡

reiterate/riˈɪtəreɪt/ v. 重申，反复说

meticulous/məˈtɪkjələs/ adj. 谨小慎微的，过度重视细节的

nucleic/nuːˈkliːɪk/ adj. 核的，核酸的

nucleic acid test　核酸检测

wreak havoc　肆虐，造成严重破坏

5.2　国外疫情防控　Epidemic prevention and control abroad①

1. 一项初步分析显示，首个有效的冠状病毒疫苗可以防止90%以上的人感染 COVID-19。

1. The first effective coronavirus vaccine can prevent more than 90% of people from getting COVID-19, a

---

① 第5.2节英文内容摘自 BBC（英国广播公司）、VOA（美国之音广播电台）、NPR（美国国家公共电台）、AP News（美联社新闻）、《纽约时报》（*The New York Times*）、《经济学人》（*The Economist*）、CNBC（美国消费者新闻与商业频道）、China Daily（《中国日报》英文版）、新华网英文版（Xinhua News）、CGTN（中国国际电视台）等网站，中文内容为作者翻译整理而成。

辉瑞和拜恩泰科将其描述为"科学和人类的伟大日子"。他们的疫苗已经在 6 个国家的 4.35 万人身上进行了测试，没有发现安全问题。

preliminary analysis shows. The developers of Pfizer and BioNTech described it as a "great day for science and humanity". Their vaccine has been tested on 43,500 people in six countries and no safety concerns have been raised.

（BBC，2020-11-09）

2. 一家领先的国际机构表示，英国将是经济受疫情影响最严重的国家之一。经济合作与发展组织（OECD）预测，到 2021 年年底，这一数字将比新冠肺炎疫情暴发前减少 6% 以上。在世界主要经济体中，预计只有阿根廷的情况会更糟。相比之下，经济合作与发展组织预测，到那时，全球经济整体将恢复到疫情前的水平。

2. The UK economy will be among the hardest hit by the pandemic, a leading international agency has suggested. The Organization for Economic Co-operation and Development （OECD）predicts that by the end of 2021 it will be more than 6% smaller than before the COVID health crisis. Among the world's major economies only Argentina is predicted to do worse. By contrast, the OECD predicts the global economy overall will be back to pre-pandemic levels by then.

（BBC，2020-12-01）

3. 法国用宵禁取代了第二次全国封锁。没有授权书，人们在 20:00 到 06:00 之间不允许外出，平安夜除外。这一规定将一直持续到新年夜。酒吧和餐馆将至少关闭到 1 月 20 日。

3. France has replaced its second national lockdown with a night curfew. People will not be allowed out the house between 20:00 and 06:00 without an authorization form. Christmas Eve will be exempt, but the rule will stay in place for New Year's Eve. Bars and restaurants are to remain closed until at least 20 January.

（BBC，2020-12-17）

4. 最近，乐购、阿斯达和维特罗斯超市宣布，他们将拒绝不戴口罩的购物者进入，医学豁免者除外。莫里森公司也采取了类似的举措，而森宝利表示将叫停那些无视规则的人。随着感染的传播，零售商被批评没有采取足够措施来阻止那些不遵守新冠肺炎防疫措施的人。

5. 美国总统乔·拜登签署了一系列行政命令，以加强与肆虐美国的新冠肺炎的斗争。美国将加快接种疫苗，并增加检测。同时，通过紧急立法以增加口罩等必需品的生产。拜登表示，战胜疫情需要数月时间，但如果人们团结起来，美国将"渡过难关"。

6. 巴西在 24 小时内首次记录了逾 4000 例与新冠病毒相关的死亡病例，因为一种更具传染性的变异加剧了病例激增。在一些城市，医院人满为患，人们在等待治疗的过程中死亡，

4. Tesco, Asda and Waitrose have become the latest supermarkets to say they will deny entry to shoppers who do not wear face masks unless they are medically exempt. It follows a similar move by Morrisons, while Sainsbury's says it will challenge those who flout the rules. Retailers have been criticized for not doing enough to stop people breaking COVID rules as infections spread.

(Xinhua News, 2021-01-13)

5. President Joe Biden has signed a raft of executive orders to boost the fight against COVID-19 which has ravaged the US. Vaccination will be accelerated and testing will be increased. Emergency legislation will be used to increase production of essentials like masks. Mr Biden said it would take months to defeat the pandemic but the US would "get through this" if people stood together.

(VOA, 2021-01-25)

6. Brazil has recorded more than 4,000 COVID-related deaths in 24 hours for the first time, as a more contagious variant fuels a surge in cases. Hospitals are overcrowded, with people dying as they wait for treatment in some cities, and the health

许多地区的卫生系统处于崩溃的边缘。该国的总死亡人数现已接近 33.7 万人，仅次于美国。

7. 人们是否愿意接种新冠肺炎疫苗，很大程度上左右着世界是否有希望回归常态，而随着这种希望的出现，专家和医疗专业人士向大家保证，还是有办法克服人们对接种疫苗的恐惧的。

8. 美国总统乔·拜登宣布采取新措施，为更多美国人接种新冠肺炎疫苗，同时批评了那些没有接种疫苗的人。总统说，大多数美国人都做了正确的事，接种了疫苗。他和他的政府对 8000 万没有接种疫苗的人感到失望。在其他措施中，他推出了涉及多达 1 亿美国人的全面联邦疫苗要求，包括命令所有员工超过 100 人的雇主，对员工提出接种疫苗或进行每周检测的要求。

9. 洛杉矶教育委员会投票决定，要求在美国第二大学区

system is on the brink of collapse in many areas. The country's total death toll is now almost 337,000, second only to the US.

（BBC，2021-04-07）

7. As the world's hopes of returning to a post-pandemic normal rests largely on people's willingness to take a COVID-19 vaccine, experts and health care professionals are assuring those people that there are ways to overcome a fear of needles.

（*The New York Times*，2021-04-01）

8. U. S. President Joe Biden has announced new steps to vaccinate more Americans against COVID-19 while criticizing those who have not gotten their shots. The president says most Americans have done the right thing by getting vaccinated. He and the government are frustrated by the 80 million who have not got vaccinated. Among other steps, he's rolling out sweeping federal vaccine requirements affecting as many as 100 million Americans, including mandating that all employers with more than 100 workers require vaccinations or weekly tests.

（VOA，2021-09-10）

9. The Los Angeles board of education has voted to require students at the age of

上课的 12 岁及以上的学生接种冠状病毒疫苗。该委员会周四的投票使洛杉矶成为目前少数要求接种疫苗的地区中最大的一个。根据洛杉矶的计划，参加体育和其他课外活动的 12 岁及以上的学生需要在 10 月底之前全面接种疫苗。

12 and older to be vaccinated against the coronavirus if they attend in-person classes in the nation's second largest school district. The board's vote on thursday makes Los Angeles by far the largest of a very small number of districts with a vaccine requirement. Under the plan for Los Angeles, students at the age of 12 and older who participate in sports and other extracurricular activities need to be fully vaccinated by the end of October.

(VOA, 2021−09−10)

10. 随着美国每天新增约 15 万例德尔塔变种感染病例和 1500 多例死亡病例，拜登上周指示拥有 100 名以上员工的企业需强制员工接种疫苗。拒绝接种疫苗的员工将每周接受新冠病毒检测。

10. With about 150,000 new Delta variant coronavirus cases and 1,500 more deaths being recorded daily in the United States, Biden last week directed businesses with more than 100 employees to mandate vaccinations for their workers. Employees who refused to get vaccinated would undergo weekly testing for COVID-19.

(VOA, 2021−09−10)

11. 总统还命令约 250 万受雇于国家政府的联邦工作人员接种疫苗，如果他们还没有接种的话。他终止了之前政府雇员可以选择不接种疫苗，而选择接受每周检测的做法。

11. The president also ordered about two and a half million federal workers employed by the national government to get the shot if they haven't already. He ended a previous option for government employees to opt out of a vaccination in favor of weekly tests.

(VOA, 2021−09−10)

12. 纽约市将要求餐馆、健身房和其他室内企业的顾客和员工接种新冠肺炎疫苗。该政策是为了鼓励更多的居民接种疫苗，因为德尔塔病毒变体正在该市和美国各地蔓延。纽约市长白思豪（Bill de Blasio）表示，该政策将"扭转疫情"。

13. 美国官员表示，从9月20日起，所有美国人都将接种新冠肺炎疫苗加强剂。疫苗将首先接种给至少8个月前接种过疫苗的医护人员、疗养院居民和老年人。白宫表示，这一举措是对德尔塔病毒变种不断上升的感染率以及疫苗保护作用减弱的证据做出的回应。

14. 美国新冠肺炎疫苗接种工作已经进入了一个新的阶段，官员们主张稳步接种加强针。目前有数百万人可以接种加强针，这些人已在6个月前接种了上一剂辉瑞疫苗。

15. 官方批准后，美国5

12. New York City is to require customers and staff of restaurants, gyms and other indoor businesses to have had COVID-19 vaccinations. The policy is to encourage more residents to get vaccinated as the Delta variant spreads in the city and across the US. Mayor Bill de Blasio said the policy would "turn the tide" on COVID-19.

（VOA，2021-08-04）

13. COVID-19 vaccine booster jabs will be offered to all Americans from 20 September, according to US officials. The jabs will first be given to healthcare workers, nursing home residents and older people who were vaccinated at least eight months ago. The White House says the initiative is a response to rising infections from the Delta variant and evidence that the protectiveness of the vaccines fades.

（VOA, 2021-08-09）

14. The United States has entered a new phase in the COVID-19 vaccination effort and officials are urging patience with booster shots. The boosters are now available for millions of people who had their last Pfizer doses six months ago.

（VOA, 2021-09-29）

15. Children between the ages of 5

岁至 11 岁的儿童将于本周开始接受新冠肺炎疫苗接种。周二，美国疾病控制和预防中心签署了这项措施。美国疾病控制和预防中心主任罗谢尔·瓦伦斯基表示，虽然儿童很少出现严重的新冠肺炎症状，但这种病毒带来的风险仍然比他们已经接种的疫苗所能预防的许多其他疾病更大。

16. 现在已经有 200 万 5 岁至 11 岁的儿童感染了这种病毒。其中 8000 多人住院治疗，172 人死亡。美国疾病控制和预防中心的独立顾问们全票支持儿童注射疫苗，称益处远远大于风险。

17. 英国政府承认无法战胜病毒，英国已经决定与新冠病毒共存，放弃与病毒作抵抗。相反，它正在研究如何最好地管理自己的存在。它的目标是保持经济开放，同时避免让医院不堪重负，近几个月来医院已经能够接受较高的确诊率。

and 11 in the United States will begin receiving coronavirus vaccinations this week after the move received official approval. The Centers for Disease Control and Prevention (CDC) signed off on the measure on Tuesday. While it is rare for children to experience a severe case of COVID, the CDC director Rochelle Walensky said the virus still posed a greater risk than many other illnesses that they are already vaccinated.

(VOA, 2021-11-02)

16. Two million children between the ages of 5 and 11 years old have been infected with the virus. Out of that number, more than 8, 000 have been hospitalized and 172 have died. The CDC's independent advisors voted unanimously in favor of pediatric vaccines, saying the benefits far outweighed the risks.

(VOA, 2021-11-02)

17. The Britain government accepts that it cannot defeat the virus. Britain is no longer at war with the coronavirus, living with COVID-19. Instead, it is working out how best to manage its presence. Its aim is to keep the economy open while saving hospitals from being overwhelmed, which in recent months has meant accepting a high

这之所以成为可能，只是因为快速且针对性强的疫苗的推广，使死亡人数保持在欧洲水平而不是美国水平，从而减轻了公众的担忧。

18. 根据英国公共卫生部的数据，免疫接种已经防止了近2500万人感染和超过11万人死亡。尽管秋季学期已经开始，而且有预测称儿童混在一起会增加感染人数，但病例数量似乎反而在下降。不过令人担心的是，病例数量冬季会再次上涨——就在医疗服务面临最大压力之时。

19. 英政府宣布对其疫苗接种计划进行调整：第一批疫苗接种将提供给12至15岁的青少年，并向脆弱人群和50岁以上的老人提供增强剂疫苗。英国这两项呼吁的发出比许多其他发达国家都要晚。

20. 政府的疫苗接种咨询委员会推迟了鼓励青少年接种疫苗的计划，理由是尽管接种疫苗对健康的益处略大于已知的危害，但不确定性高得令人

case rate. That has been possible only because a quick and well-targeted vaccine roll-out has kept deaths at European rather than American levels, dampening public concern.

(*The Economist*, 2021-09-14)

18. According to Public Health England, immunization has prevented nearly 25 million infections and more than 110,000 deaths. Despite the start of the autumn school term, and predictions that children mingling would increase infection, case numbers appear instead to be falling. But the worry is that they will rise once more during winter—just as the health service comes under the most pressure.

(*The Economist*, 2021-09-14)

19. The Britain government announced tweaks to its vaccination programme: first jabs will be offered to 12- to 15-year-olds, and boosters to the vulnerable and over-50s. Both calls were made later than in many other developed countries.

(*The Economist*, 2021-09-14)

20. The government's advisory committee on vaccination held off on recommending jabs for youngsters, arguing that although the health benefits were marginally greater than the known harms, the uncertainty was

无法接受。

21. 2021 年 9 月 13 日，鉴于新冠病毒对儿童教育和心理健康的影响，英国首席医疗官建议政府继续执行该计划。提供增强剂疫苗的决定是为了应对疫苗保护力减弱的实际情况，特别是在老年人和弱势群体中。

22. 世界卫生组织认为增强剂疫苗的接种在疫苗接种率低的国家会更有效，但英国在提供增强剂疫苗时加入了美国、德国和以色列的行列，无视了世界卫生组织的意见。以色列的早期证据表明，增强剂疫苗至少在增加保护力方面是有效的。人们希望，这些决定能够使英国避免今后的出行限制。

23. 英国政府已经重新考虑引入疫苗护照的计划。人们只是厌倦了新冠病毒强加的种种限制。然而，部长们也未选择在冬季病例上升到危险水平时要求在夜总会和拥挤的体育

unacceptably high.

(*The Economist*, 2021-09-14)

21. On September 13th, 2021, Britain's chief medical officers advised the government to proceed nevertheless, because of COVID-19's impact on children's education and mental health. The decision to offer booster shots was made in response to evidence of waning protection, particularly among the elderly and vulnerable.

(*The Economist*, 2021-09-14)

22. In offering top-ups, Britain joined America, Germany and Israel in ignoring the World Health Organisation, which argues that the jabs would be better used in countries where vaccination rates are low. Early evidence from Israel suggests boosters are at least successful in increasing protection. The hope is that these decisions will enable Britain to avoid future restrictions on behaviour.

(*The Economist*, 2021-09-14)

23. The Britain government had rethought plans to introduce vaccine passports. Persons are simply tired of COVID-19 impositions. Ministers have, however, kept open the option of requiring passports in nightclubs and crowded

场出示疫苗护照，也并未再次强制人们戴口罩并建议在家办公。但是政府的计划中没有提到过去 18 个月来一直困扰着人们的隔离。

24. 英国政府将允许一些国家的已完全接种疫苗的游客入境英国时无须隔离，已经接种了疫苗的印度人除外。上周，英国放宽了对来自 17 个国家和地区（包括日本和新加坡）的完全接种疫苗者的旅行限制，称他们在抵达英国后无须再隔离 10 天。

25. 从 2021 年 10 月 4 日起，来自这些地区的游客必须在抵达（英国）前至少两周证明自己已经完全接种了目前英国承认的新冠肺炎疫苗，这些疫苗有：牛津/阿斯利康、辉瑞-拜恩泰科、莫德纳或杨森。

26. 印度使用的疫苗主要

stadiums, and of reintroducing compulsory masking and advisory working from home, should cases rise to dangerous levels in winter. But the government's plans include no mention of the lockdowns that have plagued the past 18 months.

(*The Economist*, 2021-10-05)

24. The British government will allow fully vaccinated travelers from a list of countries to skip quarantine upon arrival, but Indians who are fully vaccinated will still need to be quarantined. The U. K. last week eased travel restrictions for fully vaccinated individuals from 17 countries and territories, including Japan and Singapore, saying they would not have to stay in quarantine for 10 days after arriving in Britain.

(CNBC, 2021-10-04)

25. From Oct. 4, 2021, travelers from those destinations would have to show that they received a full course of one of the COVID vaccines currently approved in the U. K. , at least two weeks prior to their arrival. The approved vaccines are: Oxford/AstraZeneca, Pfizer-BioNTech, Moderna or Janssen.

(CNBC, 2021-10-04)

26. India's main vaccine is the one

来自牛津大学和英瑞制药巨头阿斯利康公司，但却是由印度血清研究所以 Covishield 的名义在当地生产的，已获世界卫生组织"紧急使用"授权。

from Oxford University and British-Swedish pharma giant AstraZeneca, but it is manufactured locally by the Serum Institute of India under the name Covishield. It has been approved for emergency use by the World Health Organization.

（CNBC，2021-10-04）

27. 加拿大保守党不持反对疫苗的观点，且一直是政府采取重大行动抗击疫情的坚定支持者。但相对而言，大多数加拿大人强烈支持疫苗护照以及接种疫苗和佩戴口罩的要求。加拿大举行大选之际，新冠肺炎病例有所增加，大多数病例是未接种疫苗者，因此地方和联邦政府下令要求接种疫苗。

27. The Conservative Party of Canada doesn't hold anti-vaccine views, and has been sort of a very large supporter of significant government action to combat the pandemic. But relatively speaking, most Canadians are strongly in favor of both vaccine passports and getting vaccinated and mask mandates. Canada's national election comes as there's a rise in COVID cases mostly among the unvaccinated leading to vaccine mandates by local and federal governments.

（NPR, 2021-09-07）

28. 北马其顿一家临时成立的收治新冠肺炎病人的医院发生火灾，造成至少 10 人死亡。自 8 月中旬以来，该国新冠肺炎病例一直在上升，增加了卫生保健服务的压力。

28. At least ten people have died in a fire at a makeshift coronavirus hospital in North Macedonia. Cases of the virus have been on the rise since mid-August, increasing pressure on health care services.

（BBC, 2021-09-08）

29. 意大利从周三开始要求国内旅客出示绿色通行证，此举旨在提高疫苗接种率，并

29. Italy began requiring domestic travelers to show a Green Pass certificate on Wednesday in a bid to boost vaccinations

在有可能发生破坏性抗议的情况下限制新冠病毒的传播。该通行证能够证明，持有者在 15 天前至少接种了一剂新冠肺炎疫苗，在过去 48 小时内核酸检测呈阴性，或在过去 6 个月内曾从新冠肺炎中恢复。

30. 2020 年东京奥运会和残奥会是在前所未有的全球疫情暴发的大环境下举办的，尽管面临种种困难，但最终还是圆满落下了帷幕。

31. 为控制新冠肺炎病例激增，俄罗斯首都莫斯科开始实施新的封锁措施，只允许超市和药店这样的必需品商店营业。莫斯科乃至整个俄罗斯的疫情形势似乎都很严峻。感染病例和死亡人数都在不断上升。疫苗的接种率低是造成俄罗斯疫情恶化的关键因素，人们普遍对新疫苗特别谨慎。

32. 奥地利已对 12 岁以上未完全接种新冠肺炎疫苗的人

and limit COVD-19 transmission amid threats of disruptive protests. The document certifies that the holder has received at least one dose of a COVID-19 vaccine more than 15 days ago, has tested negative in the past 48 hours or has recovered from COVID-19 in the past 6 months.

(VOA, 2021-09-10)

30. Held against all odds under the unprecedented circumstances of a global pandemic, the Tokyo 2020 Olympic and Paralympic Games have finally come to an end.

(*China Daily*, 2021-09-06)

31. New lockdown measures have come into force in Moscow as the Russian capital struggles to contain a surge in COVID-19 cases. Only essential shops like supermarkets and pharmacies are allowed to open. It seems like a very serious situation in Moscow and across the country. The cases are going up and up, as are the number of deaths. The low vaccine take-up is absolutely crucial to this, and people are just generally rather wary of new vaccines in particular.

(BBC, 2021-10-20)

32. A lockdown has come into force in Austria for anyone over the age of 12 who

采取隔离措施。这是西欧首次对未接种疫苗的人采取此类措施。那些没有接种疫苗的人只允许离开家去锻炼、买食物和上班。

33. 在加利福尼亚的大规模核酸与早期检测系统中，加州发现了奥密克戎变体毒株。我们应假设奥密克戎也已在其他州传播。民众无须恐慌，但应该保持警惕。这意味着民众需打疫苗，去接种加强针，并且在室内也应佩戴口罩。

34. 澳大利亚国家内阁将于周二召开会议，审议旨在限制新变种传播的措施。此前，官员们进一步放松边境限制的计划暂停了两周。澳大利亚推迟了重新开放其国际边境的计划，本来还有不到 36 个小时，国际学生和技术移民就将被允许重新进入该国了。

35. 南非总统西里尔·拉马福萨表示，所有公民在回农村老家度假之前都必须接种新冠肺炎疫苗。奥密克戎变异毒

hasn't been fully vaccinated against COVID-19. It's the first such measure in western Europe for unvaccinated people. Those who haven't been jabbed can only leave home to exercise, buy food, and go to work.

(BBC, 2021-11-14)

33. CA's large-scale testing and early detection systems have found the Omicron COVID-19 variant in California. We should assume that it's in other states as well. There's no reason to panic, but we should remain vigilant. That means get vaccinated. Get boosted. Wear a mask indoors.

(Xinhua News, 2021-12-02)

34. Australia's national cabinet will meet on Tuesday to review measures aimed at limiting the spread of this new variant. It comes after officials paused a further easing of border restrictions by two weeks. Australia delayed the reopening of its international borders, less than 36 hours before international students and skilled migrants were due to be allowed to reenter the country.

(VOA, 2021-12-03)

35. South African President Cyrily Ramaphosa says all citizens have to vaccinate against coronavirus before traveling home to rural areas for the

株在南非造成了快速的社区传播，主要集中在人口最多的豪登省。

36. 世界卫生组织表示，新的奥密克戎毒株正在以前所未有的速度传播。世界卫生组织总干事谭德塞敦促各国迅速行动，控制病毒传播并保护其卫生系统。目前，该病毒变种已经在 77 个国家出现。

37. 谭德塞博士警告称，注射加强针的政策可能会再次引发疫情早期出现的问题。奥密克戎的出现促使一些国家在他们的整个成年人口中推出加强针计划，尽管我们缺乏证据证明加强针对这种变异的有效性。世界卫生组织担心，这种计划将重演我们今年看到的囤积疫苗的情况，加剧不平等现象。

holidays. South Africa has experienced rapid community spread, concentrated in its most populous province, Gauteng, which is dominated by the omicron variant.

(AP News, 2021−12−15)

36. The World Health Organization says the new Omicron variant is spreading at an unprecedented rate. The head of the WHO Tedros Ghebreyesus urged countries to act swiftly to rein in transmission and protect their health systems. The variant has now been reported in 77 countries.

(BBC, 2021−12−16)

37. Dr Tedros warned that the policy of giving booster shots may repeat the problems seen earlier in the pandemic. The emergence of Omicron has prompted some countries to roll out booster programs for their entire adult populations, even while we lack evidence for the effectiveness of boosters against this variant. WHO is concerned that such programs will repeat the vaccine hoarding we saw this year and exacerbate inequity.

(BBC, 2021−12−16)

Words & Expressions

trial/ˈtraɪəl/ n. 实验

deliberately/dɪˈlɪbərətli/ adv. 故意地，有意地（＝purposely）

conduct/kənˈdʌkt/ v. 进行，组织，实施，表现，举止，指挥，传导（热或电），带领

preliminary/prɪˈlɪmɪneri/ adj. 初步的，预备性的

humanity/hjuːˈmænəti/ n. 人类，人性，人道

overall/ˌoʊvərˈɔːl/ adv. 就整体来说（一般强调"整体"概念）

wane/weɪn/ v. 衰落，减弱，（月亮）亏；n. 变小，减弱

wary/ˈweri/ adj. 小心的，谨慎的

curfew/ˈkɜːrfjuː/ n. 宵禁

exempt/ɪgˈzempt/ adj. 免除的

flout/flaʊt/ v. 无视（规则/法律）

criticize/ˈkrɪtɪsaɪz/ v. 批评，诟病

fuel/ˈfjuːəl/ v. 推动，助长；n. 燃料

overcrowded/ˌoʊvərˈkraʊdɪd/ adj. 过分拥挤的，人满为患的

collapse/kəˈlæps/ n. 崩溃，散架

boost/buːst/ v. 推动，加强

ravage/ˈrævɪdʒ/ v. 严重破坏，毁坏

accelerate/əkˈseləreɪt/ v. 加速，加快

unanimously/juːˈnænɪməsli/ adv. 无异议地，全体一致地

pediatric/ˌpiːdiˈætrɪk/ adj. 小儿科的

emergency/ɪˈmɜːrdʒənsi/ n. 紧急事件，突发情况

legislation/ˌledʒɪsˈleɪʃn/ n. 立法

essential/ɪˈsenʃl/ n. 必需品；adj. 必不可少的，本质的

response/rɪˈspɑːns/ n. 回应，对某事做出的反应（＝in reaction to）

hoarding/ˈhɔːrdɪŋ/ n. 贮藏，积蓄，囤积

exacerbate/ɪgˈzæsərbeɪt/ v. 使恶化，使加重，激怒

inequity /ɪnˈekwəti/ n. 不公平，不公正

roll out 迁出，铺开，起床，推出

carry out 开展，实行

infect with 感染……

hold discussions about 就……进行讨论

preliminary analysis 初步分析

describe sth as... 把……描述为/看成……

safety concern 安全问题

health crisis 卫生危机，健康危机

pre-pandemic levels 疫情之前的水平

be exempt（from） 被免除（某种责任或义务）

stay in place 保持，照旧

deny entry 禁止进入

medically exempt 医疗豁免

be criticized for sth. 因为……而被指责/诟病

total death toll 总体死亡人数

turn the tide 扭转局势，力挽狂澜

a raft of 大量的

emergency legislation 紧急立法

get through 度过，熬过

5.3 疫情防控文章选摘

Selected readings on epidemic prevention and control

5.3.1 中国抗"疫"勇士 China's fighters against the epidemic[1]

文章一

击败鼠疫的中国医生

1910 年 10 月，位于俄中边境的满洲里市出现了一种神秘疾病。这种疾病传播迅速，一旦感染致死率高达 99.9%。为防止疫情向大清帝国的其他地区蔓延，朝廷派遣了出生于马来亚、受业于剑桥大学的伍连德博士北上应对。

伍博士设立了专门的隔离区，并下令封锁，以阻断感染者通行、传播疾病；他派人逐户检查，搜寻疑似病例，甚至说服俄国和日本当局于 1911 年年初的几周内彻底关闭铁路。

1910 年至 1911 年间的肺鼠疫暴发持续了近四个月，波

Article 1

The Chinese doctor
who beat the plague

In October 1910, a mysterious illness appeared in the city of Manzhouli, on the Russian and Chinese border. It spread swiftly, killing 99.9% of its victims. The Qing Imperial court had dispatched Malayan-born, Cambridge-educated Dr. Wu Lien-teh north to stop the epidemic before it spread to the rest of the empire.

Dr. Wu set up special quarantine units and ordered blockades to stop infected persons from traveling and spreading the disease. He had teams check households for possible cases, and even managed to convince Russian and Japanese authorities to completely close the railways in the early weeks of 1911.

The pneumonic plague outbreak of 1910 to 1911 lasted nearly four months,

---

① 第 5.3.1 节内容为作者根据网站资源整理而成。

及五个省和六座主要城市，造成六万多人死亡。很显然，若没有伍博士敢为人先、果断决绝地采取行动，情况也许会更加糟糕；若彼时疫情未得到控制，放任节假日期间的铁路乘客将疾病散播到中国其他地区，那么这场鼠疫造成的死亡人数将会是灾难性的，而且恐怕还会引发一场全球健康危机。

伍博士一度是世界上最著名的"鼠疫斗士"。

affected five provinces and six major cities, and accounted for over 60,000 deaths. It is clear that without the brave and decisive actions taken by Dr. Wu, it could have been much worse. Had the epidemic gone unchecked, allowing holiday rail passengers to spread the disease to the rest of China, it could have meant a catastrophic loss of life and possibly precipitated a global health crisis.

For a time, Dr. Wu was the world's most famous plague fighter.

Words & Expressions

beat/biːt/ v. 击败

mysterious/mɪˈstɪrɪəs/ adj. 神秘的

swiftly/ˈswɪftli/ adv. 很快地（=quickly）

blockade/blɑːˈkeɪd/ n. 封锁（=lockdown）

block/blɑːk/ v. 堵塞

decisive/dɪˈsaɪsɪv/ adj. 果断的

rail/reɪl/ n. 铁轨

catastrophe/kəˈtæstrəfi/ n. 灾难，横祸，困难

precipitate/prɪˈsɪpɪteɪt/ v. 引发，引起（=trigger）

beat fear 战胜恐惧

account for 导致（=cause）

go unchecked 未得到控制

a catastrophic loss of life 灾难性的死亡人数

文章二

中国"非典"战士重回公众视野，迎战冠状病毒

18 年前因抗击"非典"而家喻户晓的 84 岁钟南山院士，如今再次成为中国抗击新一波冠状病毒的公众形象。

正逢长达一周的 2020 年春节假期，新型冠状病毒的暴发让数百万春运中的中国民众惴惴不安。尽管年事已高，钟南山仍临危受命，牵头调查此次疫情。钟南山于周一宣布该病毒存在"人传人"的现象，加剧了人们对疫情的担忧。

2020 年 1 月 18 日，他从深圳抢救完相关病例回到广州，接到通知连忙赶往武汉。1 月 19 日，他实地了解疫情、研究防控方案，晚上从武汉飞往北京。1 月 20 日，他列席国务院常务会议，就如何遏制疫情扩散等提出具体建议。

Article 2

China SARS fighter returns to the spotlight in the coronavirus battle

Zhong Nanshan, an 84-year-old doctor who became a household name 18 years ago in the fight against SARS, is the public face of China's effort to control a new strain of coronavirus.

Despite his advanced age, Zhong was appointed to lead the investigation into the new virus, which has rattled millions of Chinese who are traveling for the week-long 2020 Lunar New Year holiday. His announcement on Monday that the virus could spread between humans ratcheted up worries about the outbreak.

On January 18, 2020, he returned to Guangzhou after rescuing relevant cases in Shenzhen and rushed to Wuhan upon receiving the notice. On January 19, he learned about the epidemic situation on the spot and studied the plans of prevention and control, then he flew to Beijing from Wuhan that evening. On January 20, he attended the executive meeting of the State Council as a nonvoting delegate and made specific suggestions on how to contain the spread of the epidemic.

连日来，疫情防控工作牵动人心。2020 年 1 月 20 日，钟南山出现在央视《新闻 1 + 1》视频连线中，肯定了新型冠状病毒有"人传人"现象，证实有医务人员感染，坦言人们现在对新型冠状病毒的了解还很不够，同时提醒大众戴口罩，没有特殊情况不要去武汉。十多分钟的问答，句句务实。事后不少朋友表示，直到此时才意识到疫情已悄然升级，应该提高警惕。

钟南山已经 84 岁高龄，他能够直面疫情，做出权威发言。有媒体评价，钟南山有院士的专业、战士的勇猛，更有国士的担当。

这位 84 岁的老人工作尽职尽责，为人民、为祖国、为自己肩上的责任。他尊重事实甚于尊重权威的求实精神，鞠躬尽瘁的敬业奉献精神，严于律己、宽以待人的博爱精神深深

In recent days, the epidemic prevention and control work has worried the minds of people. On January 20, 2020, Zhong Nanshan appeared in the CCTV "news 1 + 1" video link. He affirmed that someone had passed on the virus, and confirmed that there had been medical staff infected. He admitted that people's knowledge of the new coronavirus was not enough. He reminded the public to wear masks, and not to go to Wuhan unless one has a special necessary circumstance. The questions and answers lasted more than ten minutes without any pretense. Later, many friends said they did not realize that the epidemic had escalated so fast. They should have been more vigilant.

Zhong Nanshan is 84 years old, and makes a key voice facing the epidemic. He has been praised by the media for his professionalism as an academician, his courage as a soldier and his responsibility as a national scholar.

The 84-year-old man really works hard for all people and the motherland, and sees this as his own responsibility. He respects the facts more than the authority. He embodies the spirit of truth, dedication, strictness, discipline, and a merciful spirit

地打动着我们。他在疫情严峻
的形势下抵达武汉，有人称他
为逆行者，对他致以崇高的敬
意，而他则谦虚地说自己只是
一个医生！

of fraternity, which has deeply touched us
all. He arrived in Wuhan under a severe
situation during the epidemic. Some people
call him a rebel with high regards, but he is
very humble, only calling himself a doctor!

Words & Expressions

spotlight/ˈspɑːtlaɪt/ n. 聚光灯，舞台的中央（=the centre stage）

epicenter/ˈepɪsentər/ n. 中心，疫情中心

household/ˈhaʊshoʊld/ adj. 家庭的，全家人的，家喻户晓的

strain/streɪn/ n. 压力，重负，拉力，品种（动植物的）株系，类型；
v. 拉伤，损伤，使紧张，拉紧

despite/dɪˈspaɪt/ prep. 即使，尽管

appoint/əˈpɔɪnt/ v. 任命，指定（=nominate or choose）

rattle/ˈrætl/ v. 使焦虑

lunar/ˈluːnər/ adj. 月亮的，阴历的

academician/ˌækədəˈmɪʃn/ n. 院士，学会会员

pretense/ˈpriːtens/ n. 借口，（无事实根据的）要求，自称，假装

a strain of 一种（=a type of）

a strain of rice 一种水稻

advanced age 高龄

investigation into... 对……的调查

Lunar New Year holiday 春节假期

ratchet up 稳步增加（=increase steadily）

ratchet down 逐步减少

a household name 一个家喻户晓的名字

public face 公众形象（=public image）

lunar calendar 农历，阴历

5.3.2　变异毒株　Variants

文章一

德尔塔变异毒株

德尔塔变种以前被称为 B. 1. 617. 2，被认为是迄今为止传播性最强的变种，比原始毒株和在英国首次发现的阿尔法（Alpha）变异毒株更易传播。英国公共卫生官员表示，德尔塔毒株的传染性可能比阿尔法毒株高 50%，尽管对其传染性的精确估计各不相同。

德尔塔变种最早是在印度被发现的，是美国疾病控制和预防中心和世界卫生组织指定的几个"需要关注的变种"之一。它已在印度和英国迅速传播，对疫苗接种率仍然较低的地区构成了特别大的威胁。

其他证据表明，该变种可能躲过冠状病毒感染或接种疫苗后人体产生的抗体。美国疾病控制和预防中心指出，这种变异也可能降低某些单克隆抗体治疗的效果。头痛、喉咙痛和流鼻涕是目前报告的最常见

Article 1

The Delta variant

Delta, formerly known as B. 1. 617. 2, is believed to be the most transmissible variant yet, spreading more easily than both the original strain of the virus and the Alpha variant first identified in Britain. Public health officials there have said that Delta could be 50 percent more contagious than Alpha, though precise estimates of its infectiousness vary.

First identified in India, Delta is one of several "variants of concern", as designated by the C. D. C. and the WHO. It has spread rapidly through India and Britain and poses a particular threat in places where vaccination rates remain low.

Other evidence suggests that the variant may be able to partially evade the antibodies made by the body after a coronavirus infection or vaccination. And the variant may also render certain monoclonal antibody treatments less effective, the C. D. C. notes. Headaches, a sore throat, and a runny nose are now

症状，发烧、咳嗽和嗅觉丧失不太常见。

德尔塔变种还可能导致更严重的疾病。例如，苏格兰最近的一项研究发现，感染德尔塔变种的人住院的可能性大约是感染阿尔法变种的两倍。但科学家们表示，不确定性依然存在。

在美国，德尔塔变种于2021年3月首次被发现。虽然阿尔法变种仍然是美国最普遍的变种，但德尔塔的传播速度很快。美国疾病控制和预防中心的数据显示，4月初，德尔塔变种只占美国病例的0.1%。5月初，该变种占美国病例的1.3%，到了6月初，这一数字跃升至9.5%。上周，福奇表示，这个数字预计已经达到了20.6%。

德尔塔变异毒株已席卷120多个国家。现在它是印度和英国最常见的变种，占了这些国家病例的90%以上。

研究表明，尽管尚未有关于所有疫苗如何对抗德尔塔变

among the most frequently reported symptoms, with fever, cough and loss of smell less common.

Delta may also cause more severe illness. A recent Scottish study, for instance, found that people infected by the Delta variant were roughly twice as likely to be hospitalized than those infected with Alpha. But uncertainties remain, scientists said.

Delta was first identified in the United States in March, 2021. Although Alpha remains the most prevalent variant here, Delta has spread quickly. In early April, Delta represented just 0.1 percent of cases in the United States, according to the C. D. C. By early May, the variant accounted for 1.3 percent of cases, and by early June, that figure had jumped to 9.5 percent. Last week, Dr. Fauci said that the estimate had hit 20.6 percent.

The Delta variant has swept across more than 120 countries. It is now the most common variant in India and Britain, where it accounts for more than 90 percent of cases.

Although there is not yet good data on how all of the vaccines hold up against

异毒株的良好数据，但包括辉瑞-拜恩泰科和阿斯利康生产的疫苗在内的几种广泛使用的疫苗，似乎很大程度上保留了对抗德尔塔变种的有效性。

Delta, several widely used shots, including those made by Pfizer-BioNTech and AstraZeneca, appear to retain most of their effectiveness against the Delta variant, research suggests.

(*The New York Times*, 2021-06-30)

Words & Expressions

infectiousness/ɪn'fekʃəsnəs/ n. 传染性

render/'rendər/ v. 致使，造成，给予，递交，翻译，表达，粉刷

clonal/'klounəl/ adj. 无性（繁殖）系的

the original strain 原始毒株

文章二

缪变异毒株

在世界卫生组织 8 月 31 日发布的全球疫情周报中，将新冠变异病毒 B.1.621 命名为"缪（Mu）"毒株，并将其列为"需要留意"的变异株。该变异株可能具有较高的疫苗耐受性，造成免疫逃逸，因此世界卫生组织将对其开展进一步监测。

"缪"毒株于 2021 年 1 月首次在哥伦比亚被发现。哥

Article 2

The Mu variant

The World Health Organization (WHO) has designated the new Mu COVID variant, B.1.621, as "a variant of interest" that it is monitoring, according to Newsweek. The WHO said the variant has a constellation of mutations that indicate potential properties of immune escape. That means it may have the ability to evade the immunity people get from vaccines.

The Mu variant, which first appeared in Colombia in January 2021, has since been detected in over 40 countries and

伦比亚卫生部 9 月 2 日也证实，"缪"毒株是在该国发现的本土变异毒株。截至目前，已有包括英国、日本等在内的 40 多个国家和地区报告了感染该变异毒株的病例。哥伦比亚一名卫生官员称，该变异毒株于今年 4 月至 6 月在当地引发了第三波新冠肺炎疫情。

世界卫生组织声称，"尽管'缪'变异毒株在全球的流行感染率有所下降，目前低于 0.1%，但其在哥伦比亚和厄瓜多尔的流行率持续上升，哥伦比亚的流行率为 39%，厄瓜多尔的流行率为 13%"。

据美国《新闻周刊》报道，截至目前，美国共计 49 个州及华盛顿哥伦比亚特区都出现了感染该毒株的病例。美国境内只有内布拉斯加州未出现相关感染病例。加利福尼亚州共报告 384 例感染"缪"变异毒株的新冠肺炎确诊病例，为全美最高纪录，其中 167 例来自洛杉矶县。

territories including the United Kingdom, and Japan. A Colombian health official said the variant was responsible for the third surge that occurred between April and June.

"Although the global prevalence of the Mu variant among sequenced cases has declined and is currently below 0.1%, the prevalence in Colombia(39%) and Ecuador (13%) has consistently increased," the WHO said.

In the U. S. , the Mu variant has been detected in 49 of the 50 states and the District of Columbia. Nebraska is the only state not to have detected a mu variant case, according to *Newsweek*. California has reported the highest number of 384 cases, with 167 found in Los Angeles County alone.

(CGNT, 2021-09-01)

Words & Expressions

prevalence/ˈprevələns/ n. 流行，盛行，普遍，（疾病等的）流行程度

surge/sɜːrdʒ/ n. 汹涌，激增，大量，奔涌向前；v. 汹涌，使强烈地感到，激增，飞涨

constellation/ˌkɑːnstəˈleɪʃn/ n. 星座，一群杰出人物，一系列（相关的想法、事物），一群（相关的人）

immune escape 免疫逃逸

文章三

奥密克戎变异毒株

新冠病毒的新变种奥密克戎很可能会构成"非常高"的全球风险，可能在一些地区产生"严重后果"。这是世界卫生组织发出的警告，该组织建议各国加快对优先人群的疫苗接种。

我们目前了解到的是，已有13个国家报告了确诊或疑似该变种的新病例，但尚未确定的是，这一变种的传染性或危险程度如何，以及目前的疫苗对此变种的有效性。

世界卫生组织总干事表示，奥密克戎的出现意味着我们决不能放松警惕。高度变异的奥

Article 3

The Omicron variant

The new Omicron variant of coronavirus is likely to pose a very high global risk, and some regions will face "severe consequences" from it. That's the warning from the WHO's advising countries to accelerate the vaccinations of high priority groups.

13 countries we know now have reported confirmed or probable new cases of the variant, but what has not been established yet is how transmissible or dangerous it is, or how effectively the current vaccines will protect against it.

The WHO's Director-General says the emergence of Omicron means that we can't afford to let our guard down. The emergence of the highly mutated Omicron

密克戎变体的出现，凸显了我们的处境是多么危险和不稳定。我们需要的不是又一次警钟，而是应该充分认识到这种病毒的威胁。

奥密克戎变体的出现再次提醒我们，尽管我们中的许多人可能认为新冠大流行已经结束，但事实并非如此。我们正在经历恐慌和忽视的循环。来之不易的成果可能会在瞬间消失。

因此，我们最紧迫的任务是结束这种大流行病。

我们现在还不知道奥密克戎变体是否与更大的传播风险、更严重的疾病、更大的再感染风险或躲避疫苗的风险有关。世界卫生组织和世界各地的科学家正在紧急工作，寻找这些问题的答案。

variant underlines just how perilous and precarious our situation is. We shouldn't need another wake-up call. We should all be wide awake to the threat of this virus.

But Omicron's very emergence is another reminder that although many of us might think we are done with COVID-19, it is not done with us. We are living through a cycle of panic and neglect. Hard-won gains could vanish in an instant.

Our most immediate task, therefore, is to end this pandemic.

We don't yet know whether Omicron is associated with more transmission, more severe disease, more risk of reinfections, or more risk of evading vaccines. Scientists at WHO and around the world are working urgently to answer these questions.

(WHO, 2021-11-30)

Words & Expressions

consequence/ˈkɑːnsɪkwens/ n. 结果，重要性

perilous/ˈperələs/ adj. 危险的，冒险的

precarious/prɪˈkeriəs/ adj. 危险的，不确定的，不安全的，可疑的

文章四

德尔塔克戎变异毒株

一个由奥密克戎毒株和德尔塔毒株结合而成的混合变种，现在已经得到了世界卫生组织的证实。

德尔塔克戎最早出现在2022年1月，但现在已经出现了更多的病例。周三，世界卫生组织决定开始对其进行跟踪，但他们目前还没有将其定义为"令人担忧的变体"。它兼具了奥密克戎和德尔塔的一些特点。

正因如此，这一新的变种被称为"德尔塔克戎"，尽管加州大学伯克利分校的传染病学教授约翰·斯瓦茨伯格博士表示，这个名字可能会有所改变。所以这听起来是很可怕的，如果你把德尔塔毒株最糟糕的一方面——毒性更强，以及奥密克戎毒株最糟糕的一方面——传染性更强，这两者结合起来，那就会非常可怕了。

不过目前完全没有证据表明这种新的混合变种具有这两种特性。加州大学旧金山分校的传染病专家彼得·钦宏博士

Article 4

The Deltacron variant

That hybrid variant is made up of the Omicron and Delta strains, and has now just been confirmed by the World Health Organization.

Deltacron first started appearing in January, 2022, but now there have been more cases. On Wednesday, the World Health Organization decided to start tracking it, but they're not calling it "a variant of concern" just yet. It's got features of Omicron and features of Delta.

Because of that, the new variant has been dubbed "Deltacron", although Professor of Infectious Diseases at UC Berkeley Dr. John Swartzberg says that name could change. So it sounds pretty ominous if you take the worst aspects of Delta, which was a more serious illness, and you combine it with the worst aspects of Omicron, really transmissible, then you've got something that sounds pretty scary.

There is absolutely no evidence that this new recombinant virus has those qualities at all. UCSF Infectious Disease Specialist Dr. Peter Chin-Hong says both those variants were likely involved in

表示，这一新毒株的产生可能与上述两种毒株都有关。在某种程度上，如果同时存在两种流行的变体，那么实际上一个人是可以同时感染这两种变体的。不仅如此，这两种变体可以通过一些随机事件入侵你体内的同一个细胞，然后就可以开始繁衍了。钦宏博士称，在这种情况下，这一新产生的毒株就是德尔塔克戎，但他也表示，你的身体可能已经准备好对抗这一新的变种了。

到目前为止，从外表看来，德尔塔克戎和奥密克戎几乎一模一样。德尔塔克戎目前已在美国出现，但目前它还不是需要关注的头号问题。两位博士都表示，人们不应该对新冠病毒的再次变异感到惊讶或恐慌。

creating this new one. At some point, there is two circulating variants, so one person can actually catch two variants at the same time. And not only that, the two variants can invade the same cell in your body by some random event and then they can have children. Dr. Chin-Hong says in this case, those children are Deltacron, but he says your body may already be primed to fight off this new variant.

So far it seems that the outside of Deltacron is really looking almost exactly like Omicron. Deltacron has been detected in the United States, but at this point, it is not a major concern. Both Doctors say you shouldn't be surprised or alarmed to see COVID mutating again.

(WHO, 2022-03-09)

Words & Expressions

hybrid/ˈhaɪbrɪd/ n. 杂种，杂交生成的生物体，混合物，混合动力

dub/dʌb/ v. 把……称为，给……起绰号，配音，封……为爵士

ominous/ˈɑːmɪnəs/ adj. 预兆的，不吉利的

5.3.3 新冠肺炎口服药 Oral drugs for COVID-19

文章一

默克公司新冠肺炎口服药正寻求 FDA 批准通过

默克制药公司已向美国监管机构申请批准其用于治疗轻到中度新冠肺炎的药片。如果药片获得批准，它将成为第一种治疗新冠肺炎的口服药物。默克公司表示，在一项试验中，其抗病毒药物 Molnupiravir 使住院率和死亡率降低了 50%，试验对象为患有轻至中度新冠肺炎以及至少拥有一个疾病风险因素的患者。默克公司及其合作伙伴 Ridgeback 生物疗法公司已经请求美国食品和药物管理局（FDA）批准紧急使用这种药物。所有之前 FDA 批准的治疗都需要注射或静脉注射。制药商阿斯利康周一也表示，他们正在开发的一种抗冠状病毒的药物有望取得成功。阿斯利康表示，这种名为 AZD7442 的药物使非住院患者的重症及死亡人数减少了 50%。

Article 1

Merck is seeking FDA approval for its oral drug for COVID-19

Drugmaker Merck has asked U. S. regulators to authorize its pill for treating mild to moderate COVID-19. If approved, it would be the first oral edication for the disease. Merck said its antiviral pill called Molnupiravir lowered the rate of hospitalization and death by 50 percent in a trial of patients who had mild to moderate COVID-19 illness along with at least one risk factor of the disease. Merck and its partner Ridgeback Biotherapeutic have asked the U. S. Food and Drug Administration to grant emergency use of the pill. All previous FDA-approved treatments require an injection or IV. Also drugmaker AstraZeneca said Monday it is seeing promising results with a COVID-19 drug it is developing to combat the coronavirus. Known as AZD7442, the drug reduced severe COVID-19 or death in non-hospitalized patients by 50 percent, according to AstraZeneca.

（VOA, 2021-10-13）

Words & Expressions

grant /grænt/ n. 拨款，补助金，授予，给予，提供的补助金；
v.（合法地）授予，允许，（勉强）承认，同意

oral drug　口服药物

the rate of hospitalization and death　住院率和死亡率

the U. S. Food and Drug Administration（FDA）　美国食品和药物管理局

mild to moderate COVID-19　轻到中度新冠肺炎

文章二

辉瑞称其新冠口服药疗效显著

制药公司辉瑞表示，其研发用于抗击冠状病毒的实验性药物显示，如果患者足够快地服用，其因感染新冠肺炎住院或死亡的风险会降低89%。

这个结果令人震惊，该公司停止了试验，并准备向美国食品和药物管理局（FDA）申请紧急批准该药物。

辉瑞公司首席执行官阿尔伯特·博拉在一份声明中表示："今天的新闻是这一种药物能彻底制止这一流行病造成的破坏。"

Article 2

Pfizer says its COVID-19 oral medication is effective

Drugmaker Pfizer said its experimental pill designed to fight coronavirus showed an 89% reduction in the risk of hospitalization or death from COVID-19 if patients got it soon enough.

The results were so striking. The company stopped the trial and is preparing to make its case to the U. S. Food and Drug Administration for emergency authorization of the drug.

"Today's news is a real game-changer in the global efforts to halt the devastation of this pandemic," Pfizer CEO Albert Bourla said in a statement.

（VOA，2021-11-05）

Words & Expressions

hospitalization/ˌhɑːspɪtələˈzeɪʃn/ n. 住院治疗（v. hospitalize）

striking/ˈstraɪkɪŋ/ adj. 异乎寻常的，引人注目的

halt/hɔːlt/ v. 阻止

devastation/ˌdevəˈsteɪʃn/ n.（大面积的）毁灭，破坏

hospitalize sb. 送某人住院治疗

emergency authorization of the drug 药品紧急使用授权

game-changer 改变游戏的人或物，彻底改变事态发展的人、理念或事件

5.3.4 新冠肺炎疫苗 Vaccines for COVID-19

FDA 授权莫德纳和
强生疫苗允许混打疫苗

美国监管机构给莫德纳和强生加强针开绿灯，批准给接种过莫德纳或强生疫苗的美国人打新冠肺炎疫苗加强针。美国食品和药物管理局（FDA）表示，任何有资格打加强针的人都可以接种与之前不同品牌的新冠肺炎疫苗加强针。

美国食品和药物管理局大幅增加了有资格接种疫苗的人数，并在选择使用哪种疫苗作为疫苗加强针方面给予了很大

The FDA authorizes Modena and Johnson & Johnson vaccines to allow the combination of vaccines

US regulators are giving the green light to COVID-19 booster shots for Americans who got the Moderna or Johnson & Johnson vaccines. The FDA said anyone eligible for an extra dose can get a different brand than their earlier shots.

The FDA expanded the pool of people eligible for boosters big time, and it's giving a lot of flexibility in picking which vaccine to use as a booster. Anyone 65 and older

的灵活性。任何 65 岁及以上的人，如果在至少六个月前接种了莫德纳疫苗，都可以获得一半剂量的疫苗加强针；同样的情况也适用于接种莫德纳疫苗的有健康问题或者从事危险工作的年轻人，比如护士和教师；同样的情况也适用于在收留无家可归者的收容所或监狱这样危险生活环境中的人，也可以接种辉瑞公司的疫苗加强针。

对于接种强生疫苗的人来说，它甚至更加开放。美国食品和药物管理局为至少两个月前接种了本应是一针疫苗的人开了绿灯，允许他们接种全部剂量的强生疫苗。这是因为强生公司的疫苗保护力不如其他疫苗。但这是重要的一步。

美国食品和药物管理局表示，今后不一定要保持同一种疫苗接种。研究表明，莫德纳疫苗和辉瑞疫苗本质上可以作为加强针互换，这给了人们很大的灵活性，如果某一种疫苗不可用，或者人们想尝试不同的疫苗，比如说，人们第一针有不良反应。它还简化了为疗

who got the Moderna vaccine at least six months ago can get a half dose as a booster; same goes for younger adults who got Moderna who have health problems or a risky job, like nurses and teachers, or risky living situations, like homeless shelters or prisons, just like the Pfizer booster.

It's even more open for people who got the J&J vaccine. The FDA gave the green light to a full J&J dose to anyone who got what was supposed to be a one-shot vaccine at least two months ago. That's because the J&J has never been as protective as the other vaccines. But this is an important step here.

The FDA is saying that you don't necessarily have to stay in that same vaccine lane going forward. Research indicates that the Moderna and Pfizer vaccines are essentially interchangeable as boosters, and this gives people a lot of that flexibility if one vaccine is not available or if they want to try a different one because, say, they had a bad reaction the first time around. It also simplifies boosting people in nursing

养院的人们提供疫苗加强针的过程，那里的居民可能接种了不同的疫苗。这对那些接种了强生疫苗的人来说尤其重要。给强生疫苗的接种者注射辉瑞或莫德纳疫苗似乎比仅仅再注射一针强生疫苗更有利于增强免疫系统。

有些人可能仍然会再次选择强生疫苗，可能是因为这种疫苗更容易获得，也可能是因为他们更愿意获得第一次得到的东西。强生公司的疫苗在增强免疫力方面做得不错，甚至可能提供更持久的免疫力。

但有一些科学上的反对意见认为，如果人们没有变老，免疫系统没有受损，那么可能就不需要疫苗强化针了。目前还没有足够的证据证明进一步扩大强化针数量的合理性。这些疫苗实际上似乎仍然能很好地防止大多数年轻的、健康的人患上真正的疾病。但越来越多的证据表明，疫苗对一些人的保护力可能也在减弱，可能从40多岁的人开始。所以官员们表示他们将在必要时放宽资

homes where residents may have gotten different vaccines. And it's especially important for those who got the J&J vaccine. Boosting J&J recipients with a Pfizer or Moderna shot seems much better for, you know, turbocharging the immune system than just getting another J&J shot.

Some people may still go with J&J again, maybe because it's easier to get, or maybe because they're more comfortable getting what they got the first time. The J&J shot does a decent job as a booster and may even give longer lasting immunity.

But there has been some scientific pushback that if people aren't older, if they're not immunocompromized, then maybe boosters aren't needed. There just isn't enough evidence to justify expanding the pool eligible for boosters even more for now. The vaccines seem to be still actually pretty good at keeping most younger, otherwise healthy people from getting really sick. But there is growing evidence that protection may be waning for those people, too, maybe starting with 40-somethings. So officials say they'll loosen up the eligibility when that's necessary. Many people are still

格。很多人仍在等待下一次授权，为年幼儿童接种疫苗。因此，下周二，美国食品和药物管理局顾问将审查辉瑞公司授权 5 至 11 岁儿童接种该疫苗的请求。年龄较大的孩子已经在接种辉瑞的疫苗了。

辉瑞公司提交的数据显示，使用成人剂量的三分之一对 5 至 11 岁的儿童是安全有效的。如果辉瑞疫苗获得批准，这是意料之中的，美国疾病控制和预防中心将在 11 月的第一周就这个问题发表意见。孩子们需要间隔三周注射两剂，就像他们的父母一样。但这意味着许多孩子很可能在感恩节前后完全接种疫苗，这将有助于确保他们在学校的安全，并有助于防止病毒再次激增。

waiting for that next authorization for a vaccine for younger kids. So next Tuesday, FDA advisers will review Pfizer's request to authorize that vaccine for kids ages 5 to 11. Older kids are already getting Pfizer shots.

Pfizer has submitted data that using one-third of the dose grown-ups got is safe and effective for kids ages 5 to 11. If Pfizer gets the OK, which is expected, the CDC will weigh in on this question the first week of November. Kids will need two doses three weeks apart, just like their parents. But this means lots of kids could well be on their way to being fully vaccinated by around Thanksgiving, which would help keep them safe in school and help keep the virus from surging again.

(NPR, 2021−10−21)

✒ **Words & Expressions**

eligible/ˈelɪdʒəbl/ adj. 有资格的，（作为结婚对象）合适的，合格的

shelter/ˈʃeltər/ n. 遮蔽（物），庇护（处），居所，收容所；

v. 遮蔽，躲避，避难，庇护，收容所

coverage/ˈkʌvərɪdʒ/ n. 新闻报道

interchangeable/ˌɪntərˈtʃeɪndʒəbl/ adj. 可交换的，可交替的，可互换的

附录

出入境卫生检疫涉及单据

Documents for Exit/Entry Health Quarantine

附录1 出入境健康申明卡（中文版）

Annex 1 Exit/Entry Health Declaration Form(Chinese version)

中华人民共和国
出/入境健康申明卡

微信版　网页版

请在相应"□"中划"√"　□出境　□入境

姓名：＿＿＿＿＿＿＿＿＿　性别：□男 □女　出生日期：＿＿＿＿＿年＿＿月＿＿日

国籍（地区）：＿＿＿＿＿＿＿　职业：＿＿＿＿＿＿＿

1. 证件类型：□护照 □前往港澳通行证 □往来台湾通行证 □往来港澳通行证
   □港澳居民来往内地通行证 □台湾居民来往大陆通行证 □中华人民共和国出入境通行证
   □其它证件：＿＿＿＿＿＿＿＿　证件号码：＿＿＿＿＿＿＿＿＿
   乘商用交通工具出入境的人员请填写：航班（船班/车次）号：＿＿＿＿＿　座位号：＿＿＿＿＿
   *凡乘坐国际航班、列车、客车、轮渡、邮轮出入境的人员均应填写此项。

2. □境内 /□境外有效手机号或固定电话：＿＿＿＿＿＿＿＿＿＿＿＿＿＿＿＿
   其它境内有效联系人：＿＿＿＿＿＿＿＿＿　有效手机号或固定电话：＿＿＿＿＿＿＿＿＿
   境内居住地址（请详细填写，具体到街道/社区及门牌号或宾馆地址）：
   ＿＿＿＿＿省（市、自治区），＿＿＿＿＿市，＿＿＿＿＿

3. 过去 14 日内至今，您旅居的国家和地区（请具体到城市，国内地址请具体到所在街道/乡镇）：
   日期：＿＿＿＿＿＿＿＿　旅居国家或地区：＿＿＿＿＿＿＿＿＿＿＿＿＿＿
   日期：＿＿＿＿＿＿＿＿　旅居国家或地区：＿＿＿＿＿＿＿＿＿＿＿＿＿＿
   日期：＿＿＿＿＿＿＿＿　旅居国家或地区：＿＿＿＿＿＿＿＿＿＿＿＿＿＿

4. 过去 14 日内至今，曾接触新冠肺炎确诊病例/疑似病例/无症状感染者　□是 □否
   过去 14 日内至今，曾接触有发热和/或呼吸道症状的患者　□是 □否
   过去 14 日内至今，所居住社区曾报告有新冠肺炎病例　□是 □否
   过去 14 日内至今，所在办公室/家庭等是否出现 2 人及以上有发热和/或呼吸道症状□是 □否

5. 请选择过去 14 日内至今，是否有以下症状　□是 □否如有，请勾选
   □发热 □寒战 □乏力 □咳嗽 □呼吸困难 □鼻塞流涕 □头痛 □咽痛
   　　　　□胸痛 □肌肉或关节痛 □恶心呕吐 □腹泻 □其它不适症状＿＿＿＿＿＿
   过去 14 日内至今，是否曾服用退烧药、感冒药、止咳药　□是 □否

6. 过去 14 日内至今，您是否接受过新型冠状病毒检测　□是 □否
   如果您曾接受过新型冠状病毒检测，检测结果是否为阳性　□ 是 □ 否

7. 您是否曾患过新冠肺炎？　□是 □否
   如是，治愈后是否出现过核酸检测结果阳性　□是 □否

8. 您是否曾接种过新冠肺炎疫苗？　□是 □否
   如是，且已完成全程接种，完成全程接种的日期：＿＿＿＿年＿＿月＿＿日
   如您未完成全程接种：第一剂次接种日期：＿＿＿＿年＿＿月＿＿日
   　　　　　　　　第二剂次接种日期：＿＿＿＿年＿＿月＿＿日（如有）
   　　　　　　　　第三剂次接种日期：＿＿＿＿年＿＿月＿＿日（如有）

尊敬的出入境人员，根据有关法律法规规定，为了您和他人健康，请如实逐项填报，如有隐瞒或虚假填报，将依照《中华人民共和国国境卫生检疫法》追究相关责任；如引起检疫传染病传播或者有传播严重危险的，将按照《中华人民共和国刑法》第三百三十二条，处三年以下有期徒刑或者拘役，并处或者单处罚金。本人已阅知本申明卡所列事项，保证以上申明内容真实准确。如有虚假申明内容，愿承担相应法律责任。

　　　　　　　　　签名：　　　　　　　　　日期：

健康申明须知

尊敬的旅客朋友，您好！

为有效防范新冠肺炎疫情传播，保护您和他人健康，根据《中华人民共和国国境卫生检疫法》，请您按照中国海关要求，认真、如实填写《健康申明卡》，申报您的健康情况和旅行经历。如您曾在过去 14 天途经或停留过新冠肺炎疫情高发国家、地区，或目前有发热、乏力、干咳、呼吸困难等症状，请您尽早如实向机组或乘务人员报告。

根据《中华人民共和国刑法》第三百三十二条第一款的有关规定，如有隐瞒或虚假填报，造成疫情传播或有传播严重危险的，将可能被处以三年以下有期徒刑或者拘役等刑事处罚。

您可通过填写纸质版本或通过扫码"海关旅客指尖服务小程序"进行申报。抵达后，请将《健康申明卡》主动提交给海关关员，配合海关做好卫生检疫工作。

感谢您的合作！

附录 2 出入境健康申明卡（英文版）

Annex 2 Exit/Entry Health Declaration Form(English version)

 EXIT/ENTRY HEALTH DECLARATION FORM OF THE PEOPLE'S REPUBLIC OF CHINA

WeChat QR code for e-declaration

Website QR code for e-declaration

□**EXIT** □**ENTRY** (Please tick one of the boxes with "√")
Name:_____ Gender：□Male □Female.
Date of birth:_____Year_____Month_____Day
Nationality (region):_____ Occupation:_____
1. Passport No.:_____ Other identity document (please specify) No.:_____
Commercial flight (ship/vehicle) No.:_____ Seat No.:_____
  Inbound and outbound passengers taking international flights, trains, buses, ferries and cruises should fill in this item.
2. □ Chinese mobile phone/landline number:_____
  □ Overseas mobile phone/landline number:_____
  Contact persons in China and their mobile phone/landline number:_____
  Address in China (Please specify the street, community, building/house/apartment number, or the address of the hotel)_____Province (City, Autonomous Region),_____City,_____
3. What countries (regions) have you visited during the past 14 days? (Please specify the cities. For Chinese cities, please provide your detailed address.)
  Date:_____ Country (region):_____
  Date:_____ Country (region):_____
  Date:_____ Country (region):_____
4. Have you had direct contact with confirmed/suspected/asymptomatic cases of COVID-19 during the past 14 days? □**Yes** □**No**
  Have you had direct contact with people having fever and/or respiratory symptoms during the past 14 days? □**Yes** □**No**
  Has your community reported any COVID-19 cases during the past 14 days? □**Yes** □**No**
  Have there been two or more members in your office/family having fever and/or respiratory symptoms during the past 14 days? □**Yes** □**No**
5. Have you had the following symptoms during the past 14 days? □**Yes** □**No**
  If yes, please tick your symptoms with "√" □Fever □Chills □Fatigue □Cough □Difficulty breathing □Stuffy nose or running nose □Headache □Sore throat □Chest pain □Muscle pain or joint pain □Nausea and vomiting □Diarrhea □Others
  Have you taken any medications for fever, cold or cough during the past 14 days? □ **Yes** □ **No**
6. Have you been tested for COVID-19 during the past 14 days? □ **Yes** □ **No**
  If yes, is the result positive? □ **Yes** □ **No**
7. Have you been infected with COVID-19? □**Yes** □**No**
  If yes, have you tested positive for COVID-19 after recovery? □**Yes** □**No**
8. Have you been injected with COVID-19 vaccine? □**Yes** □**No**
  If yes, please specify the date when you were fully vaccinated:_____Year_____Month_____Day
  If you haven't been fully vaccinated, please specify:
  The date of the first dose:_____Year_____Month_____Day
  The date of the second dose:_____Year_____Month_____Day (if you received the second dose)
  The date of the third dose:_____Year_____Month_____Day (if you received the third dose)

Dear Passengers, according to relevant laws and regulations, for your health and that of others, please fill out this *Exit/Entry Health Declaration Form* truthfully. If you conceal or falsely declare the information, you will be held accountable according to the *Frontier Health and Quarantine Law of the People's Republic of China*, and if the spread of quarantinable communicable diseases or a serious danger of spreading them is thereby caused, you shall be sentenced to not more than three years of fixed-term imprisonment or criminal detention, and may in addition or exclusively be sentenced to a fine, according to Article 332 of the *Criminal Law of the People's Republic of China*.

I hereby certify that all the above information is true and correct. I will take the legal responsibility in case of false declaration.

Signature：　　　　　　　　Date:

The eighth edition, published on July 9, 2021

Notice

Dear Passengers,

To effectively contain the spread of COVID-19 and protect your health and that of others, according to the *Frontier Health and Quarantine Law of the People's Republic of China*, you are requested to fill out the Exit/Entry Health Declaration Form to declare your health conditions and travel history truthfully. If you have been to, either for a visit or transit, any hard-hit countries or regions during the past 14 days, or if you are showing such symptoms as fever, fatigue, dry cough, difficulty breathing, etc., please report to the crew members immediately.

According to Article 332 of the *Criminal Law of the People's Republic of China*, anyone who conceals or falsely declares the information, causing the spread of quarantinable communicable diseases or a serious danger of spreading them, shall be sentenced to not more than three years of fixed-term imprisonment, criminal detention or other criminal punishment.

You can complete health declaration either by hand writing or on the WeChat applet. When you arrive, please give your Health Declaration Form to Customs officers, and cooperate with them in health quarantine procedures.

Thank you for your cooperation.

附录 3 出入境人员填写健康申明卡指南（中文版）

Annex 3 Instructions for filling out Exit/Entry Health Declaration Form(Chinese version)

健康申明须知

　　为有效防范新冠肺炎疫情传播，保护您和他人健康，根据《中华人民共和国国境卫生检疫法》，请您按照中国海关要求，认真、如实填写《健康申明卡》，申报您的健康情况和旅行经历。如您曾在过去14天途经或停留过新冠肺炎疫情高发国家、地区，或目前有发热、乏力、干咳、呼吸困难等症状，请您尽早如实向机组或乘务人员报告。

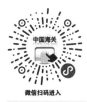

微信扫码进入

海关网站扫码进入

掌上海关（安卓）

掌上海关（苹果）

为节省出入境时的通关时间，您可使用〔中国海关互联网+网站〕、掌上海关或微信小程序，在通关前24小时内向海关申报，过关时向海关出示即可。

关于健康申明卡制度相关法律规定的介绍

一、健康申明卡制度的法律法规依据

《海关总署关于重新启动出入境人员填写健康申明卡制度的公告》（海关总署公告 2020年第16号）规定，为进一步做好口岸新型冠状病毒感染的肺炎疫情防控工作，防止疫情经口岸传播，根据《中华人民共和国国境卫生检疫法》及其实施细则等法律法规的规定，海关总署经研究决定在全国口岸重新启动出入境人员填写《中华人民共和国出/入境健康申明卡》进行健康申报的制度。出入境人员必须向海关卫生检疫部门进行健康申报，并配合做好体温监测、医学巡查、医学排查等卫生检疫工作。

二、不如实填报健康申明卡的法律责任

《国境卫生检疫法实施细则》第一百零九条、第一百一十条规定，隐瞒疫情或者伪造情节的应当受行政处罚，最高可处以一万元以下的罚款。

《中华人民共和国刑法》第三百三十二条规定，违反国境卫生检疫规定，引起检疫传染病传播或者有传播严重危险的，处三年以下有期徒刑或者拘役，并处或者单处罚金。

根据最高人民法院、最高人民检察院、公安部、司法部、海关总署3月16日联合发布的《关于进一步加强国境卫生检疫工作 依法惩治妨害国境卫生检疫违法犯罪的意见》，实施以下六类妨害国境卫生检疫行为，如果引起鼠疫、霍乱、黄热病以及新冠肺炎等国务院确定和公布的其他检疫传染病传播或者有传播严重危险的，将依照刑法第三百三十二条规定，以妨害国境卫生检疫罪定罪处罚：

1. 检疫传染病染疫人或者染疫嫌疑人拒绝执行海关依照国境卫生检疫法等法律法规提出的健康申报、体温监测、医学巡查、流行病学调查、医学排查、采样等卫生检疫措施，或者隔离、留验、就地诊验、转诊等卫生处理措施的；

2. 检疫传染病染疫人或者染疫嫌疑人采取不如实填报健康申明卡等方式隐瞒疫情，或者伪造、涂改检疫单、证等方式伪造情节的；

3. 知道或者应当知道实施审批管理的微生物、人体组织、生物制品、血液及其制品等特殊物品可能造成检疫传染病传播，未经审批仍逃避检疫，携运、寄递出入境的；

4. 出入境交通工具上发现有检疫传染病染疫人或者染疫嫌疑人，交通工具负责人拒绝接受卫生检疫或者拒不接受卫生处理的；

5. 来自检疫传染病流行国家、地区的出入境交通工具上出现非意外伤害死亡且死因不明的人员，交通工具负责人故意隐瞒情况的；

6. 其他拒绝执行海关依照国境卫生检疫法等法律法规提出的检疫措施的。

填报模版

中华人民共和国
出/入境健康申明卡

中国海关
欢迎扫码申报

请在相应 "□" 中划 "√" □出境 ☑入境

姓名：张山 　　性别：☑男 □女 　出生日期：1982 年 11 月 02 日
国籍（地区）：中国 北京 　　**常驻城市**：中国 北京 　　**职业**：教师
1. 证件类型：☑护照 □前往港澳通行证 □往来台湾通行证 □往来港澳通行证
□港澳居民来往内地通行证 □台湾居民来往大陆通行证 □中华人民共和国出入境通行证
□其他证件：_____ 　　　证件号码：EB5555555
航班（船舶/车次）号：AB123 座位号：30B 出/入境口岸：上海浦东机场 出/入境目的地：北京
2. ☑境内 / □境外有效手机号或其他联系方式：_____ 138XXXXXXXX
其他境内有效联系人及联系方式：_____ 张海 139XXXXXXXX
自今日起后 14 日的住址（请详细填写 境内住址请具体到街道/社区及门牌号或宾馆地址）：
上海市XX区XX街道XX路123号XX宾馆，北京市XX区XX街道XX路111号XX小区
8号楼1单元901室
如果属于因公来华（归国），请填写邀请方：_____ 接待方：_____
3. 过去 14 日内，您在中国旅行或居住的省（自治区、直辖市）和/或港澳台地区
（请具体到城市）：_____ 广东省深圳市、中国香港
过去 14 日内，您旅行或居住的国家和地区：_____ 意大利罗马、美国洛杉矶
_____

4. 过去 14 日内，曾接触新冠肺炎确诊病例/疑似病例/无症状感染者 　　☑是 □否
过去 14 日内，曾接触有发热和/或呼吸道症状的患者 　　☑是 □否
过去 14 日内，所居住社区曾报告有新冠肺炎病例 　　☑是 □否
过去 14 日内，所在办公室/家庭等是否出现 2 人及以上有发热和/或呼吸道症状 ☑是 □否
5. 过去 14 日内和或出/入境时，是否有以下症状： 　　☑是 □否
如勾选"是"，请选择 ☑发热 □寒战 ☑干咳 □咳痰 ☑鼻塞 □流涕 ☑咽痛
□头痛 □乏力 □头晕 □肌肉酸痛 □关节酸痛 □气促 □呼吸困难 □胸闷
□胸痛 □结膜充血 □恶心 □呕吐 □腹泻 □腹痛 □其他症状_____
过去 14 日内，是否曾服用退烧药、感冒药、止咳药 　　☑是 □否
6. 过去 14 日内，如果您曾接受新型冠状病毒检测，则检测结果是否为阳性 　☑是 □否
尊敬的出入境人员，根据有关法律法规规定，为了您和他人健康，请如实逐项填报，如有隐瞒或虚假填报，将依照《中华人民共和国国境卫生检疫法》追究相关责任；如引起检疫传染病传播或者有传播严重危险的，将按照《中华人民共和国刑法》第三百三十二条，处三年以下有期徒刑或者拘役，并处或者单处罚金。
本人已阅知本申明卡所列事项，保证以上申明内容真实准确。如有虚假申明内容，愿承担相应法律责任。
旅客签名：张山 　　日 　期：2020.03.20

2020 年 3 月 13 日，第五版

健康申明卡填报说明

一、请您如实逐项填报，如有隐瞒或虚假填报，造成疫情传播，将被依法追究相关责任。

二、第1项中，"证件类型"部分，请您在勾选您的证件种类后不要忘记填写证件号码，若您未持有所列证件，请勾选"其他证件"并填写具体证件类型。

三、第2项中，"境内/境外有效手机号或其他联系方式"应优先填写能及时联系到您本人的手机号码，若没有手机号应填写能有效联系您的其他方式。最好能填多个联系方式。

"其他境内有效联系人及联系方式"应填写您的亲属、朋友、同事或其他联系人及其有效手机号码。

"自今日起后14日的住址"应详细填写您自出境或入境后14日内的详细居住地址，境内住址应具体到街道、社区及门牌号或宾馆地址。如停留多地，请您逐一列明。

四、第3项中，"过去14日内，您在中国旅行或居住的省和/或港澳台地区"和"过去14日内，您旅行或居住的国家和地区"，如14日内旅居多地，应按照时间顺序逐一填写完整。

五、第4项中，"过去14日内，曾接触有发热和/或呼吸道症状的患者"和"过去14日内，所在办公室/家庭等是否出现2人及以上有发热和/或呼吸道症状"中的发热指的是体温大于等于37.3℃的情况，呼吸道症状包含咳嗽、咳痰、咯血、鼻塞、流鼻涕、打喷嚏、咽痛、胸闷、胸痛、气促、喘鸣、呼吸困难等。

"过去14日内，居住社区是否曾报告有新冠肺炎病例"部分，您可通过互联网、公众号等途径了解您居住社区的新冠肺炎病例报告情况后填写。

六、第5项中，"您是否有以下症状"中，请您确认自身是否有疾病症状。若有，在勾选"是"后，在症状前打勾，可复选，若症状在健康申明卡中未列举，请在"其他症状"前打勾，并填写您有的具体症状。

七、第6项中，"过去14日内，如果您曾接受新型冠状病毒检测，则检测结果是否为阳性"，如果检测结果阳性，勾选"是"，检测结果阴性，勾选"否"，若未进行过新型冠状病毒检测，可不填。

八、填报完毕后，请您不要忘记签名并填写日期。

附录4 出入境人员填写健康申明卡指南（英文版）

Annex 4 Instructions for filling out Exit/Entry Health Declaration Form(English version)

Instructions for Filling Out Exit/Entry Health Declaration Form

Notice

To contain the spread of COVID-19 and protect your health and that of others, according to the Frontier Health and Quarantine Law of the People's Republic of China, please fill out the Exit/Entry Health Declaration Form to declare your health conditions and travel history truthfully. If you have been to, either for a visit or transit, any most affected countries or regions during the past 14 days, or if you are showing such symptoms as fever, fatigue, dry cough, difficulty breathing, etc., please report to the crew members immediately.

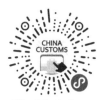

QR code for Customs services on WeChat

QR code for health declaration on WeChat

"China Customs" APP (Android)

"China Customs" APP (iOS)

To save time for passing Customs, you are encouraged to declare your health information on China Customs website, "China Customs" APP or WeChat applet at most 24 hours ahead of your travel, and show the digital bar code when passing the Customs.

Legal Basis for Filling out the Exit/Entry Health Declaration Form

I. Laws and regulations

As stipulated in the Announcement on Readopting the Health Declaration form for Inbound and Outbound Travelers issued by the General Administration of Customs of the People's Republic of China (GACC Announcement No.16 of 2020), the GACC has readopted health declaration measures to stem the cross-border spread of COVID-19 in line with the Frontier Health and Quarantine Law of the People's Republic of China, its implementation rules and other laws and regulations.

International travelers must fill out the Exit/Entry Health Declaration Form and cooperate with Customs officers on temperature monitoring, medical screening, and other health quarantine measures.

II. Legal liability for untruthful declaration

Article 109 and Article 110 of the Detailed Rules for the Implementation of the Frontier Health and Quarantine Law of the People's Republic of China specify that those who conceal or falsely declare the information will be subject to an administrative penalty of up to RMB10,000.

Article 332 of the Criminal Law of the People's Republic of China specifies that those who violate national border health and quarantine regulations, causing the spread of quarantinable communicable diseases or a serious danger of spreading them, shall be sentenced to not more than 3 years of fixed-term imprisonment or criminal detention, and may in addition or exclusively be sentenced to a fine.

According to Opinions on Strengthening Border Health Quarantine and Punishing Related Offenses jointly released by five Chinese government agencies—the Supreme People's Court, the Supreme People's Procuratorate, the Ministry of Public Security, the Ministry of Justice and the General Administration of Customs on March 16, the following 6 types of activities that may cause or risk causing the spread of plague, cholera, yellow fever, COVID-19 or other quarantinable communicable diseases identified by the State Council, will constitute the crime of impairing border health quarantine, and the perpetrator will be convicted and punished in accordance with Article 332 of the Criminal Law.

1. A person infected or suspected to be infected with a quarantinable communicable disease refuses to comply with health and quarantine measures, such as health declaration, body temperature monitoring, health assessment, epidemiological investigation, medical screening, sampling, quarantine, isolation, medical observation, on-site examination or referral, which are required by the Customs according to the Frontier Health and Quarantine Law of the People's Republic of China and other laws and regulations.

2. A person infected or suspected to be infected with a quarantinable communicable disease conceals the fact of infection by untruthfully filling out the Exit/Entry Health Declaration Form or falsifying quarantine documentation.

3. A person, who is or should be aware that microorganisms, human tissues, biological products, blood, blood products and other special articles subject to approval management may cause the spread of quarantinable communicable diseases, evades quarantine and carries/mails such articles across the border without approval .

4. When a person infected or suspected to be infected with a quarantinable communicable disease is found aboard an entry/exit conveyance, the supervisor of the conveyance refuses to follow the health and quarantine protocol.

5. When there is non-accidental death for unknown reasons on board a conveyance travelling from countries or regions with quarantinable communicable diseases, the supervisor of the conveyance conceals the truth.

6. Refusal in any other form to comply with customs health and quarantine measures that are taken in line with the Frontier Health and Quarantine Law of the People's Republic of China and other laws and regulations.

Example

EXIT/ENTRY HEALTH DECLARATION
FORM OF THE PEOPLE'S REPUBLIC OF CHINA

QR Code for e-Declaration

□EXIT ☑ENTRY (Please tick one of the boxes with "√")
Name: _____Zhang Shan_____ Gender : ☑Male □Female.
Date of birth: ___1982___ Year ___11___ Month ___02___ Day   Occupation: ___Teacher___
Nationality (region): ___China___ City of residence: ___Beijing, China___
1. Passport No.: ___EB5555555___ Other identity document (please specify) No.:_____
   Flight (ship/train) No.: ___AB123___ Seat No.: ___30B___
   Port of exit/entry: Shanghai Pudong International Airport Destination: ___Beijing___
2. ☑ Chinese mobile number and other contact information: ___138XXXXXXXX___
   □ Overseas mobile number and other contact information: _____
   Contact persons in China and their phone numbers: ___Zhang Hai, 139XXXXXXXX___
   What's your address in the next 14 days? (Please provide detailed address. For address in China, please
   specify the street, community, building/house/apartment number, or the address of the hotel)_____
   XX Hotel, No. X, XX Street, XX District, Shanghai or 8-1-901, XX Community, XX Street, XX District, Beijing
   **If you come (return) to China on (from) a business trip, please specify the inviting person
   (organization)**___XX company___ **and the host person (organization)**___XX company___
3. Where have you visited in China during the past 14 days? (Please specify the provinces/autonomous
   regions/municipalities and **cities**, including Hong Kong, Macao and Taiwan regions)
   Shenzhen, Guangdong Province; Hong Kong,SAR/HKSAR
   If you have visited other countries and regions during the past 14 days, please specify:_____
   Rome, Italy and Los Angeles, the United States
4. Have you had direct contact with confirmed/suspected/symptomless cases of COVID-19 during the
   past 14 days? ☑**Yes** □No
   Have you had direct contact with people having fever and/or symptoms of respiratory infection during
   the past 14 days? ☑**Yes** □No
   Has your community reported any COVID-19 cases during the past 14 days? ☑**Yes** □No
   Have there been two or more members in your office/family having fever and/or symptoms of
   respiratory infection during the past 14 days? ☑**Yes** □No
5. Do you have now, or have you had in the past 14 days, the following symptoms? ☑**Yes** □No
   If yes, please tick your symptoms with "√" ☑**Fever** □Chills ☑**Dry cough** □Expectoration
   ☑Stuffy nose □Running nose ☑Sore throat □Headache □Fatigue □Dizziness □Muscle pain
   □Arthralgia □Shortness of breath □Difficulty breathing □Chest tightness □Chest pain
   □Conjunctival congestion □Nausea □Vomiting □Diarrhea □Stomachache □Others_____
   Have you taken any medications for fever, cold or cough during the past 14 days? ☑ **Yes** □ No
6. If you have tested for COVID-19 during the past 14 days, is the result positive? ☑ **Yes** □ No

**Dear Passengers, according to relevant laws and regulations, for your health and that of others,
please fill out this *Exit/Entry Health Declaration Form* truthfully. If you conceal or falsely declare
the information, you will be held accountable according to the *Frontier Health and Quarantine Law
of the People's Republic of China*, and if the spread of quarantinable communicable diseases or a
serious danger of spreading them is thereby caused, you shall be sentenced to not more than three
years of fixed-term imprisonment or criminal detention, and may in addition or exclusively be
sentenced to a fine, according to Article 332 of the *Criminal Law of the People's Republic of China*.
I hereby certify that all the above information is true and correct. I will take the legal
responsibility in case of false declaration.**

Signature : Zhang Shan   **Date:** 2020.03.20

The fifth edition, published on March 13, 2020

Instructions for Health Declaration Form

1. Please fill out the Exit/Entry Health Declaration Form truthfully. If you conceal or falsely declare the information, causing the spread of COVID-19, you will be held accountable according to relevant laws and regulations.

2. Other identity document (please specify) No.: If you are holding an identity document other than passport, please specify the document type and provide the number.

3. Chinese/Overseas mobile number and other contact information: Please provide your mobile phone number. If you don't have one, please provide other contact information through which you can be reached. Please provide as much contact information as possible.

Contact persons in China and their phone numbers: Please provide the names of contact persons, such as family members, relatives, friends, colleagues, etc., and their mobile phone numbers.

What's your address in the next 14 days: Please provide your detailed address during the 14 days after you enter/exit the territory. For address in China, please specify the street, community, building/house/apartment number, or the address of the hotel. If there are more than one address, please provide them all.

4. Where have you visited in China during the past 14 days: Please specify the provinces/autonomous regions/municipalities and cities. If you have visited multiple places during the past 14 days, please specify them all in chronological order.

If you have visited other countries and regions during the past 14 days, please specify: Please specify the countries/regions and cities. If you have visited multiple places during the past 14 days, please specify them all in chronological order.

5. Have you had direct contact with people having fever and/or symptoms of respiratory infection during the past 14 days / Have there been two or more members in your office/family having fever and/or symptoms of respiratory infection during the past 14 days: "Fever" refers to the body temperature of or above 37.3 degree Celsius. "Symptoms of respiratory infection" include cough, expectoration, hemoptysis (coughing up blood), stuffy nose, running nose, sneezing, sore throat, chest tightness, chest pain, shortness of breath, stridor, difficulty breathing, etc.

Has your community reported any COVID-19 cases during the past 14 days: Relevant information is available on the Internet or official WeChat accounts.

6. Do you have now, or have you had in the past 14 days, the following symptoms: If you have relevant symptoms, please check "□Yes" and "□your symptoms". If your symptoms are not listed in the form, please check "□Others" and specify the symptoms.

7. If you have tested for COVID-19 during the past 14 days, is the result positive: Please check "□Yes" if the result is positive and check "□No" if it's negative. If you haven't tested for COVID-19 yet, you don't need to answer this question.

8. After completing the form, please sign your name with the date of signature.